Belinda Grant Viagas, N.D, D.O, Dip. C, is a trained Naturopath, Osteopath and Counsellor and has her own Natural Healthcare practice. She is the author of several bestselling books on natural healthcare, including: *Natural Remedies for Common Complaints*; *Natural Healthcare for Women*; and the *Detox Diet Book*. She is based in London and travels widely with her programme of lectures and workshops.

STRESS

Restoring Balance to Our Lives

BELINDA GRANT VIAGAS

First published by The Women's Press Ltd, 2001
A member of the Namara Group
34 Great Sutton Street, London EC1V OLQ
www.the-womens-press.com

British Library Cataloguing-in-Publication Data
A catalogue record for this book is available from the British Library.

ISBN 0 7043 4633 8

Typeset in 10.5/15 Trump Medieval by FiSH Books Ltd, London
Printed and bound in Great Britain by Cox & Wyman Ltd,
Reading, Berkshire

To dear Nora - another one!

Acknowledgements

Mary Farragher and Mary Jonmundsson ensured there were no dramas, and were senior cheerleaders, chief organisers and many other good things. Nancy Garvey was my computer pal and made learning and surfing much more fun. Raymond Harris, Baron de Vin, educated me about the stress-relieving, health-enhancing nature of good wines, and Homero Gonzalez and Steve Reid taught me how to dance Salsa. Kirsty Dunseath at The Women's Press undertook an enormous job reorganising and editing this book into its present form, and this has been further refined by Charlotte Cole.

Contents

Introduction

The stress response is your body's own best effort to save your life. It is a complex combination of physical, emotional and psychological processes that gives you the best possible chance of survival if you are being chased by a sabre-toothed tiger, or are surprised by one, who wants you for dinner. Although primitive, it is an elegant and sophisticated response that affects your whole body and your entire experience.

Nowadays, stress is a buzzword. We use it to describe our physical strains or lack of comfort, our emotional distress and life's general and specific pressures. We equate the term with negative experience. The results of long-term exposure to stress can include a range of serious conditions including high blood pressure, a compromised immune system, heart disease and stroke. Long-term exposure is the greatest single cause of ageing. It can quite literally takes years off your life.

But a small amount of stress can be a motivational force that is inspirational, galvanising our will and propelling us forward. It generates feelings of excitement, and leaves us stimulated and positive. A small amount of stress wakes us up, and sharpens the mind – we are at our sparkling best, and problem-solving skills, physical ability and sensitivity are all heightened. It adds a certain frisson to our lives and brightens our days. These good feelings can become addictive, and like any addiction we soon search out more and more of it. Increased levels of stress, however, only become damaging and destructive, robbing us of pleasure and causing us these huge health concerns.

The stress reaction was designed as a rapid response on the part of our body to anything that our mind felt we could not cope with. It is always activated according to our mental assessment of the situation. When we feel we can cope with things, we generally can, and when we feel overwhelmed, then we experience stress. Modern times see us having the same physical responses that saved our lives in the distant past, but today they still come into play when we face threats such as the humiliation of an embarrassing meeting, or the dread of sitting in the dentist's waiting room. The challenges humanity currently faces, for instance, determining new roles for ourselves and improving our communication skills (with ourselves as well as with others), seem to make little use of stress, this quite remarkable, system-wide and age-old lifesaver.

As women we face a number of specific challenges related to our gender. Each month we face the physical stresses associated with the changes of our cycle. The incidence of period 'problems' is growing extremely fast. In my natural healthcare practice, when questioned, many women will confirm that their cycle is irregular, they have cramps that are too painful, or their flow is too heavy to manage. They may also have enormous emotional and physical upheaval in the symptoms of PMS, including bloating, huge changes in appetite, alterations in sleep pattern and mental clarity and even fainting. But these are taken, somehow, as being normal – part and parcel of being a woman, and not worthy of mention unless asked. Pregnancy and childbirth take their toll on the body, and the menopause can be a stressful time. We also face extreme external stresses in trying to fit our own cyclic nature into the straight-line logic of society.

Our bodies have always been a real power base, in part because they are so intimately connected with the changing cycles of the natural world. One of the patriarchy's greatest battles with us has been on this front. Disassociating us from our body by correlating it with shame, and divorcing us from our own intimate connection with the divine have been powerful tools. The body is where we feel the attack. It is what suffers when we can no longer cope, and it is where we must begin to reclaim our own sense of self, and take responsibility for our own health and well-being.

Every day presents its own contradictions. We are the future of our species in the children that we may bear and nurture, yet this is accorded little credit, recognition or regard. Stay-at-home mums have one of the most stressful jobs – one that has little decision latitude, much psychological stress, and is highly repetitive. It has one of the highest mortality rates in our society. Career choices where we are traditionally attracted because of their versatility are usually those offering the lowest pay, benefits and social standing, and yet still have the glass ceilings and other pressures associated with women at work. We are charged with caring – to feed our babies, nurse the injured and tend to the old – but, in order to remain 'attractive' and slim, the best nutrition we can give ourselves is food which contains no calories, no goodness, no energy at all.

We are routinely overworked, underpaid and taken for granted in our working lives. A vicious cycle of poverty, under-achievement and lack of personal expression will add enormous stress to many of our lives. And in older age we can look forward to lower pensions because of the 'gaps' in our working life and our lower income.

We are repeatedly reminded of our physical vulnerability and sold the notion of our sexual availability – though the repeated pairing of sex and violence (last year in the UK an estimated 35,000 women per month were thought to have been physically attacked by their husband or boyfriend). We are encouraged to be divorced from our physicality at every turn, save for our sexual identity.

Our greatest challenge it seems is in caring for ourselves. Justifying the time to soak in a warm, scented bath without feeling guilty is vital to our long-term mental and physical well-being. Learning to value ourselves and our contribution means legitimising our own wants and needs, and expressing them.

We need to establish a strong, anchoring sense of self in order to face the world outside with all its challenges. Developing our own highly personalised stress-management programme of health-enhancing and pleasurable techniques is an investment in our own future.

The first half of *Stress*, chapters 1 and 2, is full of facts about what stress is. We look at how to recognise internal and external stresses, and positive and negative ones and there is a number of useful 'stress-busters' that can be used as immediate quick fixes when you find yourself becoming stressed.

The second half of the book, chapters 3 to 8, explores the various ways to make changes in your life in order to reduce your stress response in the long-term. This includes a review of ways to encourage deep and full relaxation; plus a look at diet, and our body's other needs. Not forgetting the mind, we examine some positive ways to think about stress as well as how to express emotions we might be used to keeping pent-up; and tips for reorganising your day to make life more streamlined.

There are plenty of ideas to choose from because it is essential for our long-term health that we find things that work for us and begin using them. This book looks at the stress in our lives from a naturopathic or holistic viewpoint – placing it in the context of our experience as women. It uses a wide range of skills and techniques that are all quite natural. They are in harmony with our being and will only encourage, enhance and support us in our move towards optimum health, happiness and vitality.

Stress is a fact of life. The challenge is how we cope with it. By appreciating the impact of stress on our everyday life, and learning to manage it, we can enjoy a more relaxed and harmonious lifestyle, feel better about and within ourselves, be able to work more effectively and better manifest our own dreams and desires. When we are not wasting our energy, we can get on with living.

Chapter 1 – What Stress Is

Stress is a complex, system-wide response to our perception. It is a complicated sequence of physiological changes that is still not fully understood, chiefly involving our hormones, nervous system and adrenal glands, and impacting on everything from how we hold our head to the rate at which we burn fat. In this wide-ranging chapter, we look firstly at the internal and external factors that can stress us and then go on to look at the stress response itself. This has three key stages – alarm, resistance and exhaustion. The hormonal changes of our menstrual cycle impact upon and are directly influenced by our stress response. Just being a woman can be stressful! Finally, we review some of the physical implications of long-term stress.

Internal and External Stress

Stressors can come from inside and outside the body. Internal stressors include our response to pain; the processing of feelings and emotions, especially the more difficult ones like fear, grief and anger; shock; our posture; and our responses to things we eat and drink. This is especially so in cases where there is heightened sensitivity or allergies to certain foods, or a depressed or depleted aspect to our digestion. The by-products of continual stress cause further internal stress if we do not allow the body time to stand down and replenish its stocks of beneficial hormones and neurotransmitters (see pp12–13).

External stress includes things that affect our environment and situations that present themselves as challenges, such as managing in relationships, handling change, and dealing with external demands such as passing a driving test or being successful in an interview. Some events can be extremely stressful, eg the death of a partner, divorce, separation, personal injury or illness, marriage, retirement, outstanding personal achievement, revision of personal habits, moving house, taking on a mortgage, holidays and even Christmas! The more stressors you have, the greater the challenge to your ongoing health.

Stress can affect us even before we are born. Research has shown that the stress hormone cortisol can cross the placenta and predispose the baby to a lowered ability to manage stress in their own life. Children who have been exposed to high levels of cortisol in this way and who have experienced stress as children are statistically more likely to experience depression and other mental difficulties later in life. This pre-birth exposure to the ill effects of stress may also contribute to the nervousness and withdrawn nature of many firstborn children.

Children who have been affected in this way may well be shy, withdrawn and inhibited, with associated health problems, such as a lowered immune response (therefore more susceptible to catching colds and flu and experiencing minor health concerns), and having allergic responses such as asthma and eczema.

It is important to remember that even good things – like falling in love, achievement and even improving our health habits – can all be stressful if only in the short-term.

Whether the source of stress is within us or outside us, our stress response is much the same. When something happens – a stimulus – we *decide* how we are going to respond to it. This is extremely important. We have a choice that is built upon our history and environment, as well as our emotional state, intelligence and what we believe to be true. We decide whether we can cope with the stimulus, or not. If we can manage, and feel in control, there is no negative stress. If we feel we cannot manage, or doubt our ability, then the alarm stage of our stress response is activated.

The Stress Response

The stress response has three clear stages.

Alarm

This is commonly known as the 'fight or flight' response, when the body is fully geared up and both ready and as able as it can possibly be to fight or flee in order to preserve your life. This is designed to mobilise all the body's resources for immediate physical activity. It is initiated by a part of the brain called the hypothalamus in response to information it receives from all your senses and the reasoning that you apply. This usually happens extremely quickly, and certainly faster than conscious awareness. The hypothalamus sends messages to the pituitary and adrenal glands to begin hormonal stimulation by a direct nerve link.

When the decision is made to stand and fight, the message from the hypothalamus is mainly to release the hormone noradrenaline. If the decision is to flee, perhaps because there is fear or uncertainty about the outcome of the challenge, then the hypothalamus signals a predominantly adrenaline release. This increases the heart rate and makes plenty of energy available for the muscle activity that is necessary to run away.

Immediate physical responses to stress:

- stress hormones adrenaline, noradrenaline and cortisol are released, which cause
- breathing to increase, and the heart to beat faster
- sweating increases
- blood is rushed to the muscles in the arms, legs and trunk
- the liver releases more sugar and fat to provide energy for the muscles
- muscles contract to prepare for sudden movement
- the pupils of the eyes dilate to ensure we take in all the information we can
- blood is diverted away from the gut, skin and kidneys – digestion and kidney function slow, and the skin may turn pale
- salivary glands dry up and the mouth feels dry.

Resistance

The fight or flight response is usually short-lived, and there are times when you may have to keep on fighting or carry on fleeing in order to save your life. This part of the stress response allows us to continue after the first rush of hormones and energy has worn off. Hormones secreted by the adrenal cortex are mainly responsible for this stage. Cortisol and its family stimulate the release of energy from protein so that the body can keep going long after the immediate glucose source of energy has burnt out. Aldosterone and its family signal the body to retain sodium and maintain an even and elevated blood pressure.

This is the part of our stress response that is engaged when we meet emotional crises and challenges, perform strenuous tasks and fight infection. It is the area where women seem to excel.

Also involved in meeting this type of demand are the hormones oestrogen and androstenedione (which is closely related to the male sex hormone testosterone). Prolonging this stage of the stress response severely increases our risk of significant disease and leads on to the final stage of exhaustion.

The main distinction we draw in terms of stressors is whether something is sudden and comes as a shock to us, or whether it is a slowly mounting and ongoing concern. We respond to shock by entering the alarm stage (as women most often manifesting the 'fear' or 'flight' side of the response) and our response to relentless stress is to linger in the resistance stage.

Exhaustion

This can manifest in the collapse of specific organs or body systems, and the earliest casualties are likely to be those areas where we have some inherent weakness, or those most challenged by the overload, eg the heart, blood vessels, adrenal glands and the immune system. The major causes of exhaustion are the depletion of cortisol and the loss of potassium ions, which destabilise the body systems. When cells lose potassium they cease to function well, and eventually just die off. When cortisol reserves are exhausted, hypoglycaemia results, and the body cells stop receiving sufficient glucose or other nutrients. That means that their energy source is non-existent.

Illnesses commonly associated with this stage include angina, asthma, autoimmune diseases (eg lupus, arthritis, multiple sclerosis), cancer, cardiovascular diseases, depression, diabetes (Type II – adult onset), hypertension, irritable bowel syndrome, menstrual irregularities including PMS and a range of more common complaints that stem from immune suppression such as the common cold, ulcers and headaches.

The Mechanisms of Stress

Our stress response is always operating – ticking over at a low rate of activity as we assess and respond to everything in our life. The daily and familiar events of our regular routine present us with demands that we know we can deal with – they pose no major threat, and we will have met them many times before. We respond to these, and to small changes in our life, quite unconsciously, activating our stress response to a mild degree without even noticing.

Unfamiliar events challenge us to make the decision

as to whether we can manage them. An area of the brain called the cerebral cortex evaluates the information that it receives from our sight, smell, hearing, touch and taste and decides what response to make. Another area of the brain called the limbic system adds emotion to the reasoning, depending on our individual evaluation of the situation. It sets the emotional tone and intensity of our decision – for instance, you may feel extremely angry about what is happening, or a little scared. A third part of the brain, the hypothalamus, deals with this joint input and – if it decides that something is a stressor – instigates a course of action in the body. There is a nervous response and a hormonal one.

A specific part of the nervous system called the autonomic branch (or division) is involved in the stress response, along with a range of hormones, of which, as we have seen, the most important are adrenaline, noradrenaline and cortisol. Oxytocin, oestrogen and other hormones also play a part.

In many respects the body is a closed unit, so what impacts upon one part will influence the whole. For instance, the emotions are stored in a part of the brain that relays information directly to the area that makes the decision about whether or not we can cope with a stress. This communication is two-way, so when we are stressed it would seem that this affects our emotional centre too. We are full of feedback loops, which means that our state can be monitored consistently and responded to instantly. Even seemingly minor alterations in anything from our blood sugar levels to our perception of the situation will bring about changes throughout the body.

The Nervous System

The nervous system is the route for the transmission of messages between the brain and the muscles, skin, organs, eyes, etc. It is in two parts. The central nervous system (CNS), which comprises the brain and the spinal cord, and the peripheral part. The CNS is split into two branches or divisions, the voluntary and the autonomic. The autonomic division has two sub-divisions that are important to the stress response: the sympathetic and the parasympathetic.

The voluntary nervous system is within our conscious control. It is the system we use to make ourselves move by sending messages from the brain to the muscles through a route of nerves that passes down the spinal column and then out into the rest of the body.

The autonomic nervous system maintains control of our heartbeat, peristalsis (the way food is moved through the gut), lung, stomach, gland and blood vessel activities. This is an area over which we have limited control, but, when our muscles need more blood to enable them to work hard, this demand is automatically met by this branch of the nervous system. It is sub-divided into the parasympathetic and the sympathetic divisions, which are a balancing and responding facility that is constantly operational, twenty-four hours a day. It is the autonomic nervous system that is most involved with the stress response. Changes in its activity produce the physical changes we need to deal with the demands we face.

The sympathetic division of the autonomic nervous system is involved in expending energy, while the parasympathetic division conserves energy. The sympathetic division is mostly responsible for initiating the stress response; the parasympathetic is involved in getting us to stand down from the stress. The parasympathetic nervous system is involved in facilitating digestion and the function of the immune system – the household jobs that are ignored when we are facing stress, yet are nevertheless essential to our continued existence.

The sympathetic system exerts a mass action throughout the body. It is fortified by the release of adrenaline from the medulla of the adrenal glands. Among its actions in response to stress are the constriction of blood vessels in the skin and abdomen, and the dilation of blood vessels in the skeletal muscles. This shifts blood from the skin and the organs to the muscles to make us stronger. Heart rate is increased, and the bronchioles dilate making it easier to get more oxygen into the body and then direct it to where it will be needed most. Digestion and urination are suppressed, and the rate of glucose release into the blood stream from the liver is increased enormously to enable us to have more energy.

The parasympathetic system's actions are more specific, and its most important actions are on the smooth muscles of the gut and the digestive glands, where it increases peristalsis and secretion of the enzymes necessary for full digestion and assimilation of nutrients.

Effects on the body of sympathetic and parasympathetic stimulus

Parasympathetic	Body area	Sympathetic
—	brain and mental activity	general increase
constriction of pupil increased secretion (tears)	eyes	dilation of pupil
increased flow	salivary glands	decreased flow
—	sweat glands	increased production
decreased rate	heart	increased rate and force
constricted to decrease air flow	lungs and bronchi	dilated to increase air flow
mild dilation throughout the body	blood vessels	constriction, excepting the supply to heart, legs and arms
—	blood	increased clotting ability
—	spleen	releases stored blood cells into the general circulation
stimulates secretion of enzymes	pancreas	lack of blood supply may diminish secretions

	gut	
increased movement		decreased activity
greater stomach acid production		less acidic stomach juice
relaxation of anal sphincter		constriction of anus
—	liver and fat tissue	mobilisation of sugar and fat stores
—	adrenal medulla	secretes adrenaline
stimulates	wall of bladder	relaxes
relaxes	sphincter	excites
erection	erectile tissue (clitoris, etc)	relaxation
—	hair follicles all over body	constriction

Most of the body is under the main control of either the sympathetic or the parasympathetic branch, although most body organs receive some messages from both branches of the nervous system. There are a few notable exceptions: the adrenal medulla, spleen and sweat glands only receive from the sympathetic division, while some of the salivary glands receive only a parasympathetic supply.

The Hormonal System

The other way to get us moving and responding to a stressor is through the hormonal system. Hormones travel through the bloodstream, each carrying a specific message. Hormones are produced by, stored in and released by glands in different parts of the body. We are familiar with some hormones such as oestrogen and progesterone, which are involved in our menstrual cycle. These so-called sex hormones and the hormones of the stress response are synthesised from the polyunsaturated fats we eat in the diet. It is the pituitary gland and the adrenal glands that are most involved in the stress response.

The pituitary is a small gland about the size of a pea that is situated in a small depression in the sphenoid bone deep inside the head. It has two parts that are quite distinct in function – the anterior and posterior lobes. Both release hormones.

The anterior lobe forms most of the gland and produces several hormones, including the human growth hormone and ACTH (adrenocorticotrophic hormone) which stimulates the growth and secretion of the adrenal cortex; cortisol (see below, p21); FSH (follicle stimulating hormone) which stimulates the ovaries and encourages oestrogen secretion; LH (leuteinizing hormone) which stimulates ovulation; and prolactin which stimulates milk synthesis and can influence the amounts of oestrogen and progesterone secretion. The posterior lobe is the storage site for oxytocin, amongst other hormones. Oxytocin stimulates the uterus to contract and milk to be ejected from the breasts. It also regulates the production of urine by the kidneys and insulin by the pancreas and influences blood pressure.

The role of oxytocin in the stress response is currently being researched more fully. It seems to be much more active as a mood regulator than we had once thought, and is involved in social interactions. Its role in the stress response is specific in that it initiates what is termed a 'tend and befriend' action in women, prompting us to reach out and mitigate some of the more depressive or internalising effects of stress. It may be that this is a quite distinct form of stress response that is unique to us, replacing or offering a viable biochemical alternative to the alarm stage. Oxytocin is also secreted by men, but seems to fail in the presence of the male sex hormones, making it more likely for them to experience a quicker and longer connection to the 'fight' response of the alarm stage. It is the presence of oestrogen – and possibly the absence of testosterone – that appears to enhance the effects of oxytocin.

There are questions as to whether and how this changes after childbirth, when the uterus has expelled its contents and the breasts are producing milk. In modern mythology, this is often a time when women become more in touch with their aggression – mainly as a protective agent to safeguard the life of their child. There are also important implications for sexually active women at different stages of their cycle.

Most of the actions of the pituitary are in response to secretions from the hypothalamus, which releases the hormones that signal the pituitary to release its own. The hypothalamus controls the secretion of adrenaline and noradrenaline by the adrenal medulla through two routes; a direct nerve pathway, and indirectly or hormonally through its action on the pituitary (via ACTH).

The two adrenal glands sit on top of the kidneys. They comprise two distinct areas: the cortex, or outer portion, that secretes principally cortisol and aldosterone; and the medulla, or inner portion, that secretes adrenaline and noradrenaline.

Cortisol has an important metabolic action essential for a normal response to stress, because it dampens our level of excitation and has strong anti-inflammatory and anti-allergy activity. (This is the base of hydrocortisone cream that is used in medicine in topical applications to soothe local inflammation.) The main job of cortisol in the stress response is to ensure a supply of fuel to the muscles that are active. It helps to convert stores of fat into available energy and, with adrenaline, it works to stimulate the action of the liver in forming glucose – another source of instant energy. Cortisol also influences brain function by blocking our access to mid- and possibly long-term memory stores. It is possible that this would be beneficial to dealing with immediate, life-threatening stress, when our need to be quick thinking and to have access to our own short-term memory stores would be paramount.

Aldosterone is involved primarily in influencing sodium and potassium excretion. This is relevant in all muscle contraction (and therefore every move we make) and also in the health of the heart. Sodium levels are especially relevant in cases of oedema or bloating and swelling due to water retention or insufficient ability on the part of the kidneys. High sodium levels help keep the blood pressure high. Too high potassium levels in the system can be toxic to the heart, causing weakness and irregularity in its rhythm. Too little potassium and cells start to die off. Aldosterone is the most active substance known to promote sodium retention, and has important clinical applications. It is intricately involved in the maintenance of a good electrolyte balance.

Androgens are also secreted by the adrenal cortex. These are steroid hormones that produce masculine signs in excess, and are associated with the strength of our libido. They are produced in minuscule amounts here, and also by the ovaries.

Adrenaline is produced by the adrenal medulla. It is a different type of hormone from those produced by the adrenal cortex, being protein based and synthesised from the amino acid tyrosine, as is noradrenaline. The medulla usually secretes about four times as much adrenaline as noradrenaline. Both of these support and prolong the sympathetic nervous system's stress response, their major effects being on the heart and lungs, and on the metabolism. They increase the heart rate and the force of the beat, and enhance the blood vessels in muscles, constricting those in the skin and the abdomen. Noradrenaline is a vasoconstrictor, constricting the blood vessels, and adrenaline is most potent as a stimulator of the heart. Both hormones stimulate the process of glucose production and the mobilisation of essential substances from fat deposits. The release of glucose from the liver means a sharp rise in blood sugar levels and lots of instant, available energy. These two hormones bring about essentially the same results as the actions of the sympathetic and parasympathetic nervous system (see table on pp17–18).

People commonly speak of feeling the adrenaline flowing when they begin to feel energised and start to appreciate some of the stimulating and positive effects of stress. Actually it is *noradrenaline* that is responsible for arousal, increased physical strength and the feelings of excitement and drive. It stimulates special areas in the brain that produce feelings of pleasure, and it is the 'high' or the 'buzz' to which we can become quite addicted.

The feelings of having high circulating levels of adrenaline are actually quite unpleasant. This is the hormone that is responsible for the desire and the ability to run away, and is likely to make you feel slightly sick in your stomach, very over-stimulated (like having had too much caffeine) and somewhat scared.

The link between hormones and feelings and emotions is apparent, but there is much more research to be done before we know the full picture. There is still much to learn about just how effectively a feeling can trigger a hormone, and vice versa. What is clear is that we can change the way we feel through the power of our mind, and that this will have a hormonal effect on the whole of the body, reinforcing our feelings. It is also clear that the current hormonal balance of our body directly affects our feelings and emotions. When we feel anger and aggression (the fight response), it is due to increased levels of noradrenaline. There is also a small increase in adrenaline and androstenedione levels, but little change in the levels of cortisol. When we experience fear and a sense of withdrawal (the flight response), we have high levels of adrenaline, there is a small increase in noradrenaline, and cortisol levels increase. Depression and submission occur in the presence of raised levels of cortisol, but there is little or no change in the others, save for a small drop in androstenedione. When we feel quietly or serenely happy as in relaxation or meditation, both noradrenaline and adrenaline levels fall, and there is little or no change in the others. Feelings of elation such as those when we are on a high, and feel loved and secure see androstenedione levels rise, and everything else fall.

The Menstrual Cycle

Each month our internal and external climate, and our responses, go through tremendous change. Usually the hormonal changes finesse together quite seamlessly making for an even, roughly 29-day cycle, but sometimes this doesn't work too well and violent symptoms and mood swings occur. The very changes throw up their own stresses, imposing a greater load on our inner homeostatic ability. Trying to ignore the power of this cycle with all its fluidity and change, and fit into a linear, non-changing, logical way of being can put tremendous strain on us.

The changing hormonal picture that governs our menstrual cycle is directed by the pituitary gland in response to the directions from the hypothalamus, in much the same way as the stress process. If there are insufficient resources, it is always the more vital of these processes – the life or death stress process – that will take precedence. Lack of periods is a classic sign of long-term stress.

The menstrual month can be split into two distinct phases: pre-ovulation and post-ovulation when fertilisation or a period will result. During the pre-ovulation phase when oestrogen levels are rising, our hormonal balance sees us being more outgoing and positive; at and after ovulation, when progesterone levels are highest, we experience energy peaks, and feel at our most confident, energetic and capable. As these hormone levels change leading towards menstruation, we become progressively more inward-looking and reflective.

The intimate links between oestrogen levels and noradrenaline are yet to be fully researched. Studies on menopausal women suggest that hot flushes are related to noradrenaline metabolism in the absence of oestrogen, which dampens its effects. At menopause a whole reorganisation of the neuro-endocrine system occurs, with the adrenal glands taking over production of oestrogen precursors (substances that the body can use to convert into oestrogen). The commonly accepted symptoms of the menopause are most likely to be due to adrenal depletion (as a result of long-term stress); high levels of noradrenaline that is still in the system; and an absence of seamlessness in the conversion and change of use within our endocrine system. One of the most common causes of menopausal difficulties is due to the shrinking and exhaustion of the adrenal cortex from continued cortisol exposure. High levels of noradrenaline lead to increased calcium loss in the urine, which can cause, or certainly exacerbate, osteoporosis.

Positive Stress

We need a certain amount of the energy that comes from our stress hormones in order to lift us beyond the boredom and frustration of being under-involved. When we have too few demands upon us we can also experience the stress of feeling that we are wasting our time and we need some degree of pressure to arouse us!

A certain amount of stress can be motivating, exciting and inspiring, adding a frisson to otherwise mundane situations and times. It can spur us on to achieve great things, providing a sense of challenge. Creativity, efficiency and effectiveness are all associated with the positive effects of stress. This is achieved when we feel we can handle a situation or a potential stressor or stimulus, and our stress response is activated within a normal, balanced zone. Enough stimulation is received in order to pep us up a bit, without tipping over into a full-scale alert.

Noradrenaline increases our alertness, improves our concentration, sharpens our mental ability, and enhances both our learning and decision-making abilities, and it makes us feel good. Keeping in a positive stress situation means encouraging a small amount of noradrenaline, but not experiencing the adrenaline-associated symptoms of feeling awful, forgetting things, and having reduced concentration and decision-making skills. We do this by keeping the demands that we perceive as being placed upon us within a manageable range, and by building our store of coping skills and resources.

The size of our zone of positive stress is unique to each one of us, and will change through our monthly cycle and in response to a whole range of other life events. The better we feel within and about ourselves and our skills and ability to manage in the world, the more we are able to keep stress in our positive zone (or within our own personal stress threshold). The way to remain in this realm of positive stress is to reduce or limit the pressures we experience, and to build our reserve of coping strategies, memories and techniques. It is important not to become addicted to the positive aspects of stress. It feels very good to be motivated and effective, and the danger is that we want more and more of that feeling – stretching ourselves beyond our own reasonable limits. The key to continued good feelings is therefore to increase and enhance our ability, not to search out more of the same stimulus.

Negative Stress – Physical Concerns

Of course too much stress does affect us negatively. The ill effects of stress are likely to be felt in the body systems that are most affected by the sudden changes and shifts in energy that the response involves, and also in the areas where we may have any inherent weakness or face constitutional challenges. Some of the specific health concerns associated with overexposure to stress include heart attack and stroke, blood pressure problems and the myriad effects of having a weakened immune system.

The major work of noradrenaline is to constrict blood vessels during the alarm stage of the stress response, and this increases the pressure of the blood, meaning the heart must work harder to circulate it. Noradrenaline also increases the heart rate, so there is tremendous pressure on the heart, and it needs more oxygen and glucose in order to meet these demands. These are delivered by the coronary arteries.

The coronary arteries are prone to partial or complete obstruction by plaque in a condition called atherosclerosis. When this occurs, the heart may not be able to receive the supplies it needs in order to meet its workload, and the pain of angina can be felt as a pain across the chest, often in response to increased exercise or an activated stress response. More severe is a heart attack, when a sudden and severe reduction in the blood supply leads to the death of part of the heart. If only a small part of this magnificent muscle is affected, life can continue and the heart bears the scar. This is the case for about half of those who experience a heart attack. For the rest, a heart attack is usually fatal.

There is some research to suggest that noradrenaline can rupture plaque deposits. This is very dangerous and allows blood clots (also enhanced by the action of noradrenaline) to form and cause blockages at the site from which they have ruptured. Angina and heart attacks can also occur even without coronary artery disease (although it has been estimated that most of us in Western society have some degree of this due to our high-fat diet and low exercise habits), when noradrenaline causes the arteries to spasm and constrict, restricting blood passage.

When the stress hormones work together to mobilise glucose and fat stores and provide extra energy, they raise the levels of glucose, cholesterol and fats in the blood. High circulating levels of cholesterol are another high risk factor for coronary heart disease because cholesterol is a major component of plaque. Whatever cholesterol is eaten has an effect on blood cholesterol levels, but much more is released into the blood stream as a result of the stress response than could ever be eaten in one meal. High levels of noradrenaline and adrenaline in the blood may also cause damage to the inner lining of the blood vessels, which allows plaque formation.

When there is additional fat in the blood stream, the blood becomes thicker, and requires the heart to work harder in order to pump it around the body. This is further complicated by the thickening of the blood due to the spleen releasing its store of red blood cells into the circulation. When this happens in large amounts, the blood can become extremely viscous and may block some of the smaller blood vessels. If this happens in the heart, a heart attack is likely. If it happens in the brain, it will cause stroke.

Excessively high levels of noradrenaline also have a direct effect on heart muscle, reducing its ability to beat.

The role of sodium and potassium balance is extremely important. Aldosterone is responsible for increasing the body's retention of sodium and the excretion of potassium. High sodium levels will maintain high blood pressure. Low potassium levels lead to physical exhaustion. When body cells lose potassium they initially function less effectively, and then die.

The heart can suffer interruptions and insult silently

and without the dramatic pain of angina or the collapse of a full attack. Silent heart attacks can be experienced with very few associated symptoms, but the heart may well become weakened as a result of them. The silent attacks vary from an abnormality in the heart rhythm, to a full ventricular fibrillation. This is when the main chambers of the heart lose their basic rhythm, and the heart cannot beat effectively. A major cause of these silent heart attacks is stress, and there appears to be a strong indicator that repressed emotional stress is a major trigger, although further research needs to be done to confirm this.

Heart disease is the greatest single cause of death among women – five times as many die from heart disease as from breast cancer, and twice as many as from all cancers. It kills more women under 65 than anything else. We are still less likely than men to be suspected of heart disease or even heart attacks, and we receive far fewer referrals than men to cardiac specialists.

Heart concerns manifest differently in women, and the symptoms we need to look for include:

- chest pain that builds up slowly, starting as a niggling ache or concern (rather than the crushing immediate pain pattern that is common to male heart attacks)
- tiredness
- shortness of breath.

Our hormones play a major role in the condition of our heart, changing as we pass through the menopause and leading us towards greater risk of heart disease as oestrogen levels in the body decline. Until then it has a protective effect. While menstruating continues, there is also the possibility of angina that is related to the cycle. Research is currently being undertaken to confirm that attacks peak at the end of each cycle, although some studies show peaks mid-cycle.

The subtle energy of our heart – the emotional centre of our being – is tried enormously throughout our lives, as we struggle to have our feelings and emotions acknowledged and respected.

It is not just the heart that can suffer. Persistently high blood-sugar levels can lead to pressure on the pancreas and possibly to diabetes. This is more likely if there is a history of it in the family. The effect of stress on digestion is enormous. Eating, processing or assimilating our food while digestive ability is suppressed can cause problems anywhere along the length of the gut. In the stomach, more acid is produced during the stress response, but the effect of cortisol means the healing process that works on the walls of the stomach is dampened, so indigestion and even stomach ulcers can occur. When we are not fighting off bacterial invasion, from the food we eat, we are more vulnerable because of the effect of cortisol.

The nervous stimulus we experience during the

stress response encourages the bowel to remain closed, and peristalsis is reduced, so there is the potential for constipation and all its associated health concerns – piles locally and malabsorption of essential nutrients on a more general level.

When energy is diverted away from the reproductive system on a long-term basis, we can experience a lack of sexual responsiveness, interrupted menstruation and lowered fertility. Stress not only upsets our hormonal balance, but also causes contraction of the Fallopian tubes and reduces the blood supply to the pelvis. It can inhibit the proper development of the lining of the womb and lead to vaginal spasm and the full range of menstrual irregularities. Emotional factors figure large for us in this area, and their involvement in the activation of the stress response cannot be overlooked. When we feel negative or fearful about this aspect of our lives, it can initiate the stress response.

When we experience chronic, long-term stress, endorphin levels – the feel-good chemicals in the brain – become depleted, causing our resistance to pain to be lessened as well as our ability to feel good within and about ourselves. Persistent or unrelaxed muscle tension can exacerbate existing complaints such as arthritis and can also lead to back and neck pain, headaches and migraines.

Not all of us who experience stress will experience life-threatening diseases, but we are all likely to experience some degree of distress, or some compromising of our health and well-being, if our stress levels are not managed effectively. Not all of the health concerns outlined here are caused solely by our stress response, but it does have an impact on our constitution, and can exacerbate existing conditions.

Many of us will experience some of the more common early symptoms of adrenal exhaustion – low circulating hormone levels and increased anxiety. We may also notice insomnia; appetite changes; mild depression; loss of interest in things generally, and specifically in ourselves, in our social and other relationships and in sex; and other sub-clinical complaints such as tiredness, lethargy, mild skin complaints and headaches. In general, stress-related symptoms are likely to increase in severity the longer we are under stress. It is not possible for us to see many of the effects of stress, such as our blood clotting more easily, or more red blood cells being pumped into the blood stream. Some signs are very clear, however, and it is essential that we become adept at spotting them. These are explored in the following chapter.

Chapter 2 – Recognising and Managing Stress

Each stress response is individual, because it is activated directly by our own unique assessment of the stimulus. The more accomplished, confident and in control we feel, the less likely we are to experience the negative aspects of stress. It is also true that the more we express our feelings, emotions and pent up physical energy, the less likely we are to suffer from the more negative side effects of long-term stress. When we are able to control our own inner responses, we can also control the rise and fall of our stress reaction.

First of all we need to know how and where it is that stress affects us most, and what it is that specifically stresses us. Then we can learn how to catch it early before it builds into a problem, and will know where to target our relaxation and other techniques to best effect. The relaxation response (see pp75–76) is diametrically opposed to stress, and when we use it both as an instant fix and as part of continued lifestyle management we re-educate ourselves at the most basic level of response. In this chapter, we will see how to recognise our own unique stress response. We look at the three main personality types to see which response is most like our own and how we might like to change it and then take a look at where we hold our stress physically. Finally, there is a variety of quick-fix remedies to manage our reaction on an everyday basis, until the long-term strategies in the next chapters take affect.

Recognising Stress

Personality Types

Some of us enjoy a challenge, and feel stimulated by the prospect of change and excitement. There are those who actively seek out thrills and risks, undertaking challenges that others wouldn't even consider. And some of us seem to naturally value constancy, commitment and calm above all else. The first type has become known as Type A personalities, the risk seekers as Type T and the more mellow as Type B. This rather mundane nomenclature came about as the result of an early study into the effects of stress on men with heart problems. The group observed was of high-risk men and it was called group A in the research, and the naming has stuck.

Type A people try to squeeze the maximum from their day. They will talk faster in order to save time, eat quickly to let themselves get on with the next thing, and walk quickly in order to get there faster. They will always endeavour to do more than one thing at once, juggling seemingly unrelated tasks, and often being successful in all of them. These are the classic workaholics, who have short fuses, short attention spans and few creative outlets.

Type B people tend to be much less driven, although they can still experience great ambition and success. Their approach tends to be very different. They do not panic, lose their temper or operate on a constant high-energy level. They are also very good at giving attention to all the areas of their life such as families and friends, and will express themselves creatively and enjoy their leisure. Commitment to all areas of their life is a source of satisfaction to this type, they tend to have belief in their own ability to effect positive change in their lives, and view challenge as normal.

Type T people are easily spotted. They hang-glide, go parachuting and bungee-jumping. They are the extroverts in every group, and appear to thrive on stress. They are remarkably resilient to the long-term effects of stress. This appears to be a fairly new type of stress response and is being studied to see the full chemical profile. It is possible that this is an adaptation in response to our current environment where stress is not necessarily life-threatening, but may in fact enhance our experience.

Type As are more prone to stress-related illnesses and worries. Early on they can show the positive sides of stress, like having great energy and facing each new challenge with renewed vigour. Prolonged exposure to stress can result in them becoming more hostile and viewing new challenges as a threat that must be bested.

Check the following list for Type A behaviours that you recognise in yourself and those close to you:

- finding fault with other people
- constantly criticising others
- overly competitive at work, at home, in games, with the TV, etc
- habitually late for appointments
- always doing things in a rush
- quick to anger over small things
- easy to anger with yourself if you make a mistake
- doing several things at the same time while working out what you will be doing next
- lack of patience, even with trivia such as while waiting in queues or in traffic jams
- take little time to relax
- have few outside interests
- can become obsessive over minor detail
- often finish other people's sentences in your impatience to move along.

Many of these behaviours can be un-learned, and the result is a calmer and happier outlook, and the prospect of a much healthier future. Revisiting the quality of relationships, enjoying yourself and having a good laugh regularly, looking after yourself and expanding your interests, can all have hugely beneficial results in reducing your stress and increasing your life satisfaction. Chapters 3 to 8 suggest where in your life you can make these changes.

There are other ways to classify ourselves. Different personality types will seem more vulnerable to the ill effects of stress by manifesting the symptoms in distinct ways or areas of the body. Some of us are thinkers and worriers, for example, while others tend to hold and experience the ill effects of stress as a build-up of physical tension and unexpressed energy. Where we experience our vulnerability to stress is where the symptoms of stress-related illness are likely to show.

Some of us quite naturally seem to respond to stress by coping with it. These people are calm in the face of all life's challenges, seem to find the time to think through what the next step should be and are confident that they will survive. They are flexible and consider all the options to any given situation. These are the people that others count on.

Some of us crumble and find that just about everything is a catastrophe or a crisis. Nothing is straightforward, and the worst almost always seems to happen. They make mountains out of molehills whenever there is an opportunity to do so.

Most of us are quite capable most of the time. We may find that we cope with some situations, but crumble in others. It is important in managing your stress levels that you trust your own intuition and strength, so thinking through all those times in the past when you have triumphed over difficulty and managed your life well will always help. Remember those personal skills and techniques that you have used to be successful in the past, and remind yourself of them often.

Some of the different responses to stressful situations that we find ourselves in include:

- Feeling the need to take control. This is a typical type A response.
- Worrying and fretting, and having a delayed response. This is a more typical response to the long-term effects of stress, and when we do not feel we have control over our lives.
- Being a drama queen and using the excitement as a distraction from on-going stress. These people enjoy the racing pulse and the pounding heart that just add to the thrill of the moment.
- Erupting like a volcano with angry outbursts that often need a victim to be let loose upon.
- Playing possum – becoming ineffective and doing nothing – but the body will often respond by fainting,

feeling dizzy or just being overwhelmed by events.

Ideally, most of us would like to be situation reactive – blasting our way out of threatening situations like a volcano when that is needed, and riding the waves of excitement when it is safe enough to do so.

Stress Audit

- Audit your day and define those areas that present the greatest challenges. Note where you feel able to meet them successfully, as well as those parts where you actively experience some degree of negative stress. If you feel uncomfortable considering an area, it is likely to be a source of stress!

- There are a number of common, everyday occurrences that can be mildly irritating when they happen to us as a one-off, but when they seem to occur all the time they can tip us over the edge into a very real stress response. Consider factors such as being late for things, or being kept waiting, feeling let down or disappointed by people, experiencing personal rudeness or being ignored. Look also at the things you do quite naturally – perhaps multi-tasking, or other long-established habit patterns – in relation to every area of your life to see if these are still as positive and effective in your life today as they once were. Treat this as a serious task, and one that you need to do in order to fully appreciate, and begin to remedy, any negative effects that the stress response may be manifesting in your life.

- Ask yourself some of the following questions:
  - what things make you smile?
  - when did you last compliment or praise someone close to you?
  - are you enjoying your life?
  - do you spend enough time with your family?
  - when did you last enjoy an evening out?
  - do you feel guilty when you make time for your own pleasure?
  - can you spend money on yourself?
  - are you expressing your creativity and experiencing your own view of the world?
  - do you feel good in your body?
- It is also good to try to identify your own prime stress. We can usually identify one thing in our lives that is a major source of stress, and that could be improved or altered in some way in order to improve the quality of our life. This might be something as seemingly generalised as 'other people' whose arrogance or superficiality constantly confound you or it could be the very specific fact that you can't drive and so are always dependent upon others whenever you need to travel anywhere. This is as a major project to which you can apply your own best problem-solving skills, imagination and ingenuity in order to change your prime stress into something

more manageable (also see Setting Realistic Goals, p195).

- Think for a few minutes about the last time you were aware of the feeling of being pressured or stressed. Think about the sort of things that troubled you, and the situations in which you felt tense. Which relationships make you feel tense? Are there any places or environments that evoke a stress response? List as many of these as you can.

- It is important to notice where you feel the symptoms of the stress response in your own body. This will help you target those areas with relaxation and other techniques. It could be that you always notice a bit of a stomach ache once you start to wind down from a stressful situation, or you could be aware that you are grinding your teeth, swinging your leg, tapping your feet, or employing other displacement activities such as pencil tapping, nail biting, etc.

- When you review those situations and things that affected you, try also to recall whether you were aware of any emotional change. Did your mind feel clear? Ask yourself how clearly you are able to remember the situation or event in all its detail. Did time seem to pass by slowly, or had it speeded up? Was your sleep troubled? What other things do you notice?

Record this information so that you can refer to it later, and use it as a benchmark for future change.

Spotting the areas in which you felt stressed may not be very easy if you are not used to identifying your own stress response. Look over your day with a view to seeing how easy you felt all the time, how happy or able to smile you were, and how you responded to those around you. If you can't remember smiling at all, maybe you had a thoroughly stressful day. Other things to look out for include: times when you were aware of your heart beating; or that your breathing felt shallow and your muscles tense; or you felt like you wanted to cry, scream, or throw something; or when you felt impatient, irritable and anxious. You may experience stress more subtly as an absence of creativity or sexual interest, or an increased incidence of minor accidents, or in making silly mistakes.

It may help to look in a mirror and assess your posture – see if your fists are clenched, if your jaw is loose, and whether your neck muscles are too tight, throwing your head back slightly and making you look as though your shoulders are hunched. Note which habits cause discomfort.

Some of us respond to stress with increased mental energy, some with a peak in physical energy, and some on an emotional level. It is quite common for us to feel easiest with one of these areas of expression, and that is likely to be the area where we most notice our stress. This is important because this is where we need to direct our most active relaxation skills. It also sheds light not only on our inherent strengths, but also by relief on those areas of our life which could be further developed in order to balance our experience.

Body Scan

This is a powerful technique for identifying where you are holding stress and tension in your body right now. Take a few minutes to do this body scan and then record your findings. You will be able to identify and then write down the areas that are your own current tension spots. This is going to become your own personal checklist of places to watch out for. Once you know if you hold your tension in a specific area of your body, you can start to use the instant physical relaxation exercises on pages 53 to 60.

Set aside ten minutes when you will not be disturbed, and sit comfortably. You are going to scan through your body with your imagination. Close your eyes and take a deep relaxing breath. Breathe out slowly, and feel yourself settle and become comfortable in your own energy. Do this a few times. Now, with your imagination, scan your left foot and see whether there are any areas there that are painful, tight, cool or tense. Work your way slowly up your left leg, scanning all the time, until you reach your hip. You don't have to do anything, just notice any spots that don't feel relaxed. Now check out your right foot, and work slowly up your right leg to your hip, scanning and noticing all the time. Take your time, and stay relaxed about this – all you are doing is taking a look to see what your body is holding.

Scan your way up your body now, moving through your pelvis and up towards your neck. Notice if there are any areas that are painful or tense. Move to your left shoulder, and check how tense it is, then move down your left arm and into your hand. Notice where your areas of tension are – which finger is the most tense? Now scan your right shoulder, and then down your right arm and into your hand, checking all the time to find out whether any areas are holding tension. Then move up your neck and all around your head and your face noticing where there is tightness.

At the end of your body scan take a few more deep, relaxing breaths before you open your eyes and slowly and gently stretch out your arms and legs, as though you are just waking up. Take your time, and when you are quite ready, write down or record those areas where you noticed tension. Common sites are the forehead and jaw, neck and shoulders, stomach and bottom, but tension can be stored anywhere in your system. As you remember and record each location, return to it for a moment with your awareness so that you can reinforce your memory of it. It may be that the area will feel lighter or looser, or more relaxed, because sometimes just attending to an area and recognising it will be enough to let it relax.

Breathing Patterns

We breathe all the time, so often assume there is nothing to it – certainly nothing that we might need to practice. Check out your current breathing pattern – it is likely to change dramatically depending on how relaxed you are. For instance, when we are emotionally distressed we tend to hold the area around our heart tight, so breathing remains shallow and confined to the upper chest.

Sit comfortably and attend to your breath. Notice if there is a regular pattern to it, and whether it feels smooth and easy. Is it fast or slow? Where does your breath go – high into your chest or deep down into your belly? Does it flow easily into and out of your body? Just listen for a while and see. Check it too at various times in your day – especially when the pace steps up – and see what happens then.

Ideally, your breathing pattern wants to be deep and full, comfortable and relaxed. See pages 80 to 85 for some relaxation exercises connected to breathing.

Making a Body Map

This is a wonderful way to develop a better relationship with your body, to feel easier and more comfortable within it. It will connect you with the feelings and emotions that you have and that affect you physically as well as on a more subtle level – setting up a physical or emotional predisposition. It can be very enlightening if you didn't record any physical symptoms on your stress audit or if you noticed that many of your stressors had an emotional component.

This exercise requires a little forward planning. You need to do it with someone else who will read the directions for you and take notes of what you say. Make some time when you know you will not be disturbed, and be sure to turn off the telephone, or take whatever actions are necessary to ensure a quiet and peaceful time for yourself.

Lie down and make yourself comfortable. You can lie on a bed, but on a mat or quilt on the floor is better because you will be relaxing quite deeply and don't want to fall asleep. You can also lie on a sofa if this is easier, or on a treatment couch. Make sure that you are warm and that your back and head are well supported. Begin by taking some deep, easy, relaxing breaths and close your eyes. Now breathe in deeply, and as you breathe out, imagine any stress and tension leaving your body, being carried out on your breath. Do this a few times, then make your breathing a little more relaxed, and a little slower. Do not strain, but let your breathing deepen and relax you even further. Become aware of feeling warm and supported and how safe and secure this is.

Have the person you are working with begin naming parts of your body, one at a time, and then writing down whatever you tell them about it. Consider this list:

Chin

Left leg

Left arm

Bottom

Nose

Tummy

Abdomen

Tongue

Forehead

Left foot

Heart

Shoulders

Hair

Hips

Womb

Right arm

Inside head – your brain

Pelvis

Right leg

Chest

Neck

Genitals

Right hand

Right foot

Throat

Ears

Eyes

Left hand

Mouth

Lips

Anywhere else that hasn't been mentioned.

As you hear each body part suggested, just wait and see what happens. Sensations, feelings, images or other messages will come to you. Just relate them out loud so that you will be able to review them later. Don't work to try to understand them or interpret them at this stage, just be relaxed and receptive, and see what comes. Some of us have very good visual skills and may see picture images, others might feel sensations such as coolness or be reminded of a scene or an aspect of the natural world, or words might come to mind. If nothing comes to you at all in response to a suggestion, that is fine too. Simply give yourself a little time to be sure, and then move on.

One patient of mine who did this exercise kept saying 'Nothing's coming' after each body part. We worked through almost half her body with the same response, but I noticed that she kept screwing up her eyes. I asked her to tell me just what she was looking at and she said that it was like sitting in front of the TV, and that the screen was right in front of her, but it was blank. I suggested that she look for the power switch, which was at the bottom of the screen, and turn it on. After that she saw very clear visual images projected onto the screen. At the end of the exercise, she switched off the monitor, but she returns to it for relaxation or whenever she wants to reconnect with her body-self in this way.

The last item on the list is 'anywhere else that hasn't been mentioned'. This is an important moment to see whether your body has any other message for you, or if there is any other area that needs your attention. After this, just relax and lie still for a few more minutes, before slowly starting to come back to your everyday reality.

Take a few big, deep breaths, and as you exhale wriggle your fingers and toes. With the next exhalation, gently stretch your arms and legs. You will have been relaxing quite deeply, and want to be gentle with yourself. Roll over onto your side if this is more comfortable, and take as long as you need before getting up.

Now you can review what came to you as you worked through the different parts of your body. You might also like to make a physical map of your body – get a friend to trace your outline on a large sheet of plain paper (the back of a sheet of wallpaper is good). You can write, draw or colour in the areas to record your findings. Take some time to interpret any symbolism that you uncovered, and to comprehend the full value of your understandings. Whatever jewels of self-knowledge you have uncovered in this exercise will be a great store that you can return to whenever you need reassurance about your feelings, the connectedness of your experience, or your progress. You may also see how things change for you by returning to this exercise in the future.

Managing Stress

There will always be things in our life that we experience as stressful and there are real benefits to be gained from managing our stress levels well. We can maximise the positive experience of increased focus, galvanised intention, a clear mind, physical impetus and heightened problem-solving ability. Stopping this from spilling over into the more negative effects of stress requires us to be aware of what is happening in and around us, and to have our own range of resources for coping with the stress we experience. In the long-term, this means maintaining optimum health and well-being through a lifestyle that is supportive; prioritising sleep, rest and renewal, and keeping diet sharply in focus. In the short-term, we need to develop a resource of fast-acting remedies to set off our relaxation response as soon as we notice ourselves becoming overly stressed.

Positive Influences

This is especially important at times when we experience greater stresses, larger expectations than usual, or are going through change. Even beneficial change is a challenge that can require us to access our own deeper resources in order to maintain equilibrium. There are some factors that positively influence our ability to manage a range of stresses, and research shows that the following impact directly on our ability to cope:

- having supportive family and friends
- being involved in a social or activity group
- having a hobby or other creative pursuit
- taking regular exercise
- having some daily spiritual practice or meditation or experiencing the relaxation response (see pp75–6)
- having somewhere that you can be on your own
- taking time for yourself to do things that you enjoy
- having a sense of spiritual connection
- being able to give

- keeping a pet, or having access to one
- regular satisfying sex.

The greater the love, support and positive encouragement we receive from those around us, the lower our stress response, and the better our overall health. Research also shows us that the more able we are to express ourselves, and the more fulfilled our experience of life – the more satisfied we are with both ourselves and the way we live – the less likely we are to experience the problems of negative stress in the long-term.

Taking Instant Action

There are times when we can feel the unpleasantness of rising stress levels. Even if you are just beginning to uncover your own personal response to stress, there are some situations that will stand out. It may be that you experience frustration, anger, or fear in circumstances that are not life threatening and would be resolved more beneficially if you retained control. Generally speaking, if you lose control then you won't be able to influence what is happening enough to ensure both your own safety, and a successful outcome. Gaining control of some aspect of what is going on will enable you to feel more secure, and give you time to put your coping mechanisms into play. It will also relieve you of a great deal of the pressure and negative feelings that come with being powerless.

Obviously, there is a definite limit on what you are able to control or influence in any physical situation, but while you are in it, you will still be able to work with your own emotions and responses. This is when knowing the quick fixes that work best for you can save both your own health and the situation.

The most important thing you can do in any situation is to know what you want. If you stay centred in yourself and in the present you will be able to react and become responsible (able to respond), rather than just reacting. Our instincts can be lifesaving, but often we will be just reacting to other people's agendas, and it is important to establish our own. Preparation, and thinking through different scenarios so that you are more ready to meet them, will stop you from being caught off guard, and may allow you to positively influence both your experience and that of others who are involved.

Sometimes just taking a breath will be enough to buy you a moment of time in which to reconnect with your own inner sense of calm. This will also start to relax you. Easing any physical tension will almost always help. Whenever possible breathe out as slowly as possible, and for as long as possible. (This is like the 'counting to 10' advice with which we are almost all familiar.)

Relaxing key muscle groups that you know you tense will often stop stress from building. For instance, an early sign can be when the muscles at the back of the neck constrict enabling the head to lift and see further, which is great if we are in physical danger but less than useful otherwise. Consciously relaxing the neck muscles (see pp63–5) will reverse the process. (See also Using an Anchor on p93 to help with emotional distress.)

Expending physical energy is always a good stress-buster. Simply getting up and moving will often be enough to relieve physical stress as well as changing the dynamic of any situation.

Try the following techniques to find which work best for you. When you find one that works, use it – commit it to memory and use it whenever you need to.

Being Real

Sometimes just acknowledging what you are feeling is enough. So, if you are sitting in the dentist's waiting room and you really feel like running away, acknowledge it. Think through the possibilities. Say to yourself, well, I could run away, it's what I feel like doing.

Opening a dialogue like this lets your brain assist rather than setting up a split between what you think and what you feel. It will also help you feel more in control of the situation and, as we have already seen, that is an important aspect of managing your own stress levels.

Accept that you feel like running away, and think

through the consequences – you might have to re-book or cope with some toothache. But be open to the messages that your body is sending – maybe this anxiety is just about this particular dentist and you need to find another one.

You can also use this in relationships with others – telling the other person what is happening, eg 'I am finding this extremely frustrating,' or 'I am becoming angry and so I am going to bring this conversation to an end.' See also Chapter 7, Emotions and Feelings.

Four Steps

1. Take a deep breath. This will help settle you and give you the energy and clear-headedness you need to approach the matter sensibly. It will also buy you a moment of time.
2. Do a reality check. Name in your mind five things that you can see around you, eg the window, the door, etc, or repeat your name, the date, your age, the season and where you are physically right now, eg I am in the garage.
3. Register your feelings. Acknowledge if you are feeling uncertain, angry, anxious or fearful.
4. Decide what it is that you want to happen. Endeavour to achieve the best possible outcome for yourself in this immediate situation. If you can determine what that is, then you will know what you need to do next.

Stop

If you are aware that your stress levels are rising because of the way you feel or because you can tell that a situation is escalating, say sharply and distinctly to yourself 'Stop!' Say it out loud if you can, otherwise say it clearly in your own mind.

Then take a deep breath in and hold it for a moment before breathing out, as slowly as you can, relaxing your shoulders and your hands while you do so. Then take another breath in and as you breathe out relax your forehead and jaw.

Carry on with what you were doing but make your movements smoother and slower, and, if you are talking, speak more slowly with your voice pitched a little lower than usual.

Five Point Plan

1. Close your eyes if possible, and focus on whatever is causing your stress or annoyance. Be as specific as you can, really pinpointing the stressor.
2. Repeat out loud or inside your mind 'My mind is alert, my body is calm. This is not going to get to me.'
3. Smile. This is important because it sets up a relaxation response, relaxes your forehead and jaw, and repeats to your body the message that you have just spoken or thought. Practice an inner smile so that you are able to replicate it on occasions when it would not be appropriate to smile openly.

4. Breathe in to the count of three
5. Breathe out to the count of five.

Circular Breathing

This is a wonderfully restful and centring exercise that can be used for just a moment or two when you need an instant calmer – just before going into an interview or after a scary event – or that can become a regular part of your relaxation programme. Like many exercises, it might look quite complicated on a first reading, but once you have practised you will be able to use this as an instant and very effective tool to relax and centre yourself.

Sit, stand or lie down comfortably, and place the palm of your left hand over your belly button. Cover this with your right hand, and relax your shoulders. Take a few deep, relaxed breaths, and let your hands focus your attention so that you are breathing right down into your belly, and then right out from there. Picture in your mind the place just below your belly button that is the centre of your body and a rich resource of vital energy. See your hands acting as a filter or protector for this vital place.

Now, take a deep breath in, and picture yourself breathing right into this area, and as you breathe out, let your breath come from there too. Count to four in your mind as you breathe in, and then hold your breath for a count of four. Breathe out while you count to four, and then stay empty to a count of four. Then breathe in again to a count of four, and carry on the cycle. Keep your counting slow and relaxed and maintain the pace throughout all four directions of the circular breath. Try not to speed up, force your breath or gasp for air – get the speed of your count so that the whole thing is comfortable and relaxing. Keep breathing this way for as long as you like, until you feel quite settled.

Instant Relaxation

Breathe in to the count of three, and imagine that the air is coming into your body through holes in your feet. Feel the sensations of fullness and warmth spread all the way up your body, ending at your head.

Breathe out to a count of three and imagine your breath leaving your body, draining down from your head and out through the holes in your feet. Feel how full and warm your body is. Relax your muscles, and let your jaw and your shoulders go limp. Repeat three times, or more if necessary.

Standing Relaxation

This is one of my favourite exercises which you can either do in an instant or take your time over. You can use it to start any relaxation, exercise or meditation session. It can be done anywhere without drawing much attention to yourself, and I find it most useful when there is a build-up of physical tension, or when you have to stay still for any length of time. It owes much to the Pilates system of body control.

Stand with your feet a little apart – hip-width is good. Imagine three points on the soles of your feet – one at the base of your big toe, one at the base of your little toe, and the third in the middle of your heel. Your weight wants to be evenly balanced between the three. Once you are stable, let your knees soften, relaxing them slightly and letting go of tension in your thigh muscles.

Draw your belly button in towards your spine and at the same time imagine a small weight dropping down from the base of your spine, lengthening and straightening it. Let your breastbone go soft, and lengthen the space between your shoulders and ears. Really relax your shoulders and arms and feel all the joints loosen. Lengthen the back of your neck, and straighten your head so that your chin is parallel with the floor. Imagine that there is a large bunch of balloons attached to the top of your head, lifting it up and away from your neck.

Good posture is not static, so do not try to hold this position by force, just enjoy the feelings of being balanced, but lighter and more relaxed.

Relieving Postural Tensions

How we feel within and about ourselves will have a big impact on our posture and how well we are able to deal with the stress we encounter. When we feel down, or tired, or undervalued, we tend to slump our shoulders, take smaller steps, and let our head hang down a little. When we feel inspired and loved and fit and sexy we walk with attitude, holding our heads up and moving more quickly. Once you know this, you can act your way into feeling better. Holding your usual 'feel-good' posture will remind you of what it is like to feel great, and has a de-stressing effect even when you are not feeling great. This works because your body is full of feedback loops, and if the information coming into your brain from your muscles and the proprioceptors in and close to your skin is that you are moving in a relaxed and confident way. This will positively influence your decisions about becoming stressed.

Other factors influence our posture too. Women with big breasts may experience shoulder and neck strain, and lower back problems. A well-fitting bra and extra attention to developing abdominal and shoulder muscles will help. Fat women place a lot of stress on the spine unless their abdominal muscles are good and strong. The biggest impact on our structure comes from what we wear. Even the shape of the shoes we wear often bears no resemblance to the natural shape of our feet, and this can cause muscle problems in the hip and thigh area as well as sore feet. The spine is a stack of bones that fit together one on top of another in a gentle sequence of curves. When we wear high heels we throw that balance right off, and if we then put a heavy bag over one shoulder we create a series of postural challenges that are complex and can be difficult to deal with. Repeating this pattern every day can create real, deleterious change in the spine and throughout the rest of the body.

Good posture is easy and relaxed, and enables your body to work at an optimum. It naturally releases muscle spasm and makes sure that no new tensions or stresses are created.

Instant Postural De-stressing

- Always push your bottom to the back of your seat so that the very base of your spine gets some support.
- Relax your jaw muscles right now, and let your chin drop back a little, so that your head actually drops forward slightly. Most heads weigh around 14lb and need to be carried well if they are not to tax the neck and shoulder muscles.
- Take a deep breath.
- If you are standing still for any length of time, shift your weight from one foot to the other, or support first one foot then the other on a step, low shelf, or pile of books. (Remember this the next time you do a household task like ironing or washing up for more than five minutes.)
- Don't stay in the same position, seated or standing, for more than 30 minutes – get up and walk around the room to relieve your postural muscles.
- Keep your tools at the right height – adjust your keyboard and screen so that you can reach and use

them comfortably and make sure your chair and desk height suit you; raise or lower kitchen surfaces, etc.

- Watch yourself in a mirror to see how symmetrical your posture is – do you habitually hold your head on one side, or always have one shoulder higher than the other? These postural habits can often be unlearned, or may respond to gentle correction from a practitioner. (Consult a naturopath or other natural healthcare practitioner who uses osteopathy, cranial osteopathy, cranio sacral therapy, or a chiropractor or Alexander teacher.)
- Do not hold the phone between your ear and your shoulder. If you use the phone a lot invest in a headset.
- Make sure your bra is professionally fitted. Tight clothing restricts blood flow and increases tension in the muscles and a badly fitted bra will only create discomfort.

Relaxing Your Shoulders

Try these exercises to see which ones suit you best, and then use them every day until you re-learn how to do things without tensing your shoulders. Ask yourself, too, what it is that you are bearing the weight of – heavy responsibilities, a duty of care, the burden of others' expectations? Working on lightening these loads may help your physical tension.

- Sit comfortably, and close your eyes. Imagine a huge cloak of rich, thick velvet being placed lovingly around your shoulders. See the beautiful colours, and how it shines as the light catches it, and feel its warmth, and the way that its weight draws your shoulders down. Relax into the good, warm feeling that embraces you, and take three deep, relaxing breaths while you enjoy it.

- Take a deep breath in and draw your shoulders up as high as they will go. Hold them there for a count of five, and then breathe out to a count of eight and slowly lower your shoulders as you count. Repeat three times.

- Massage the muscle along the top of each shoulder with your opposite hand. This is a long muscle that stretches down your neck and out towards your shoulder socket. Be gentle but firm as you use your fingers and thumb to almost lift the muscle, stretching it and then letting it lie back again.

- Keeping your back straight, slowly drop your head forward until your chin is sitting on your chest. Place your hands very lightly on the top of your head, and relax them. As the elbows come down, the weight of your arms will slightly but effectively stretch the muscles in the back of your neck and relax your shoulder girdle. Take easy, deep, relaxed breaths, and do not make any sudden movements – keep it very fluid and slow-moving. You will feel your head dropping still further until you reach a natural conclusion. Then slowly lift your hands off, and slowly straighten up your head again.

Relaxing Your Stomach

Stomach tension is a little harder to spot than raised shoulders. Clues are if you notice that: your breathing is very shallow; your torso feels fixed, rigid, or not as flexible as you would like; and having food intolerance of some kind. Two questions to ask yourself are whether there are things that you don't want to take in any more, and whether you feel vulnerable or in need of strength. Good exercises include:

- Breathe right out as far as you can, then draw your belly button in, as though you are trying to make it touch your spine. Hold for a count of five, then slowly release as you take a new breath in. Repeat this two or three times.
- Sit comfortably, and close your eyes. Take a deep, relaxing breath and imagine a ball of glowing, strong light right in the middle of your body. See how strong it shines, and how its radiance reaches out to every part of you. Concentrate on the very middle of this and gradually work on strengthening the colour until you have at your centre a sun that glows with a strong, nurturing, golden yellow that is the brightest thing in your universe. Let yourself

bask in the warmth of its glow for a while, before opening your eyes. Return here for some very personal sunbathing as often as you are able.

- Go somewhere that you will not be disturbed, and stand or sit with your back straight. Give voice to the whole energy of your body using the sound OHM. This is an ancient word for peace, and it has been used for centuries in spiritual and meditation practices. Its sound, and the individual sounds that comprise it, resonate to different parts of the body and the energy that we hold in these sites. Begin this by opening your mouth wide, and feeling the full, round aao that begins at the very bottom of your belly coming up through your body and changing as it reaches your middle into a more aow sound, then up through your heart area and up into your head until it becomes the more closed-mouth hum. You will need to tighten your abdominal muscles to move the energy up and out through your mouth. Do this slowly and quietly to begin with, and repeat several times. It is very energising and you will need to take a moment afterwards to settle yourself before getting on with your day.

- Practise pushing out with your tummy muscles in short, quick movements. Push against your waistband, or against your hand, or stand up against a wall. Breathe out before you start, and then push out with your tummy several times as quickly as you like, before taking a new, full, deep breath in. Repeat this three to five times.

Relaxing Your Bottom

This is a common site for muscle tension. It is one of the largest muscle groups in the body, and also a spot where fat deposits. Tension here can lead to a range of physical complaints including constipation and impaired digestion. It can also become a reservoir for emotional energy that it is difficult to let go of, or to express creatively. If this is where you hold your tension, ask yourself what it is you need to release in order to move on in your life. This can also point to you needing to ground yourself more, and to be able to get to the bottom of things. Help this part of you relax by:

- Tightening the muscles in and around your bottom so that you actually sit up a little in your seat. Hold them tensed for the count of five, and then relax them and take a deep breath in. Do this three to five times whenever you think of it, or make it part of a routine to do it every time you sit down, or on the hour, every hour. This is an isotonic exercise.
- Go flamenco, salsa or merengue dancing. These styles all focus on this area – Flamenco encourages you to stamp out any tensions as you use precision and care to place your whole body weight.

Merengue is very good for loosening up your back and ensuring a good flow of energy through your spine. Salsa is all about controlled leg and hip movements and is just about the most fun you can have in public!

- When you walk, use shorter steps that usual. This tones the muscles in the upper leg and the bottom. Target this area with specific exercises and general measures such as climbing stairs, and walking with your heels lower than the ball of your foot, to increase tone.

Relaxing Your Fists

When you are under stress your body will habitually adopt certain poses, often without you being fully aware of it. Clenching your fists, or holding your thumb inside your fingers are both clear signals from your body that you are feeling under pressure. Make it a part of your general relaxation to check on the state of your hands regularly, and to relax them just as often. Sometimes you will notice this tension in terms of gripping your pen really tightly, or taking too firm a hold on anything from your child's hand to the newspaper you are reading. Other clear hand signals that your body uses are picking at your nails, playing with your hair, and twiddling your thumbs.

You can use this energy in different ways by playing with a set of worry beads, or using your hands to do different things, such as intricate work or something that requires strength. There are also executive toys, and small rubber balls that you can play with to release some of the pent-up energy. Most effective of all though is to use the state of your hands as an indicator of the amount of tension you are currently experiencing and use it as a cue to consciously relax.

Do these hand exercises when you have a moment:

- A good first exercise is to spread your fingers out wide, stretching them as far as you can to make a wide span, and then curl them up quickly into a tight fist. Repeat this quickly about five times to awake the energy flow to your hands and leave them feeling a bit lighter and looser.
- Shake your hands, holding your arms steady and letting them move freely from the wrist. Shake them up and down, then from side to side, quite fast. Do this for at least one minute to start them tingling. Then rub the palms of your hands together as fast as you can for about half a minute. When you stop you should feel them to be warm and toasty, and almost glowing with energy.

When you have done your exercise, let your hands go quite limp, and cradle one with the other as you relax for a moment.

Tools That Can Help

There are a number of tools that can help as effective stress remedies. Some people benefit from wearing a gemstone or a piece of crystal to change their energy and help calm and ground them. Quartz crystal is naturally settling if you can find a piece that resonates with your own energy. Rose quartz is linked specifically to emotional calming and topaz to mental clarity.

You might also be interested in the effects of electro-magnetic devices. These have long been used for diagnosis and treatment and can now be used by individuals. They can be very effective in raising your stress threshold, and improving your general health and vitality, and it is now possible to wear a form of miniature ceramicised magnet that is wonderfully safe and effective. This is an excellent and completely non-invasive way to alter your whole body chemistry, stabilising cell activity and helping your muscles stay relaxed. This can also work wonders to relieve period pains as well as supporting long-term relaxation. (See the Resources for more details.)

There are many 'anti-stress' devices on the market, including a special tool that shoots streams of very low level electricity to electrodes clipped onto your ears. This is thought to 'retune' the neurones in your brain that are wound up through anxiety.

Flower remedies are another soft and gentle way for

helping to deal with life's emergencies, as well as with more general ongoing stress. They are especially effective on the subtler levels such as our feelings and energy levels. There is a wide range available, including the Dr Bach range which uses flowers common to the UK and Europe. They are made by containing the active principles of the flower within a solution of water or alcohol. Good remedies for dealing with stress from the Dr Bach range include Rescue Remedy which is a composite remedy that acts to calm, soothe and settle the system; Holly to help with the alarm stage, making it easier to manage; and Olive to help restore reserves of energy. There is a wide range, so you can make your own choice based on the literature available and your own experience. To take, put a few drops into a glass of water and sip slowly, or place the drops on your wrist or other pulse point for your body to absorb. If you are worried about the alcohol, add drops to a glass of hot water and leave to cool before taking. Take as often as you feel you need to until you feel calm.

Long-term Care

Once we have met the immediate challenge with a successful coping mechanism or technique, we need to continue shaping our lives and balancing periods of stress with periods of calm. Experiencing the relaxation response (see pp75–6) builds a resource of good memories in the muscles and the mind that will have an ongoing positive effect in terms of keeping us calm in times of rest as well as helping us to stand down from stress.

A lifestyle that is responsive to our changing needs is necessary in order to deal with long-term stress. We need to be able to know our own optimum sleep needs, and keep to a timetable that works for us in order to provide a solid framework to our days. When the situation demands it, the use of deep relaxation techniques and meditation can augment our ability to adapt. Ongoing good nutrition means we are more able to meet demands successfully, as well as having both the energy reserves and the dietary resources to rise to the physical challenge of whatever stresses we face.

The following chapters explore a range of resources that all form part of our armoury against the negative effects of stress. They include things we might consider to be treats, but they are not at all – rather they are essential to our being able to maintain our overall and everyday effectiveness. The best remedy of all is always the one that we enjoy, and the delight of the following chapters is that so many of the ways that we may reharmonise and balance our lives are so enormously pleasurable.

Chapter 3 – Relaxation

There are many different ways to relax and settle ourselves. For some people, simply switching off from immediate concerns or leaving them behind as they walk out of the door is enough. The rest of us need to practise these skills, and we can all benefit from relaxation techniques that work for us. The best results will always be gained through regular practice, and the effects are cumulative, so these efforts are well rewarded. Spending just 10 minutes each day on practising and enjoying being relaxed has been shown to produce real benefits in stress reduction.

Having used some of the quick fixes in the last chapter for responding immediately to a stress response, we can now look at more ongoing or longer-term strategies for coping. Many of these skills and techniques can be refined and adapted to fit into your own schedule once you become familiar with them. Do not be tempted, though, to skimp and save time by doing any of them quickly, or less than thoroughly. And do not try to avoid making some special time for yourself each day when you can legitimately relax and do nothing else.

Smile!

The most valuable thing you can learn to do to relieve your stress levels is to smile. Having fun, enjoying yourself and laughing are the best and cheapest stress-busters you will ever find. When you crack the mood and stop taking yourself and life quite so seriously you open the door to some real relaxation, and a deep healing. Just smiling means you produce more antibodies in your system to improve your immune system and increase your energy levels. Having a good laugh means giving your body a full massage from the inside, as well as being one of the most pleasurable activities we know.

Become Your Own Best Friend

Taking time to regularly be on your own will enable you to relax and replenish your energies, and be more able to give yourself to your relationships with others. This can take the form of a short time each day when you practise a relaxation technique, or regular 'away-days', or a monthly retreat.

Looking after yourself – placing your own physical and emotional health on a high priority rating – means you are more likely to feel able to justify to yourself taking time and doing the things that you know are good for you. Becoming your own best friend means you will be more able to lavish love and respect upon yourself.

We all have an intuition, so cultivate your own inner voice and listen to it. It will be your best guide when things become busy or confusing, and can draw your attention to the areas of your life where you need to tackle stress, and the areas of your body where its ill effects are proving problematic.

The Relaxation Response

The relaxation response is a specific physical and emotional event that is diametrically opposed to our stress response. We can practise it and learn to experience it to counter the negative effects of stress. This goes beyond the relaxation we may gain from sitting in front of a fire, or reading a book or sleeping, and is designed to give a specific effect.

When we experience stress, the sympathetic nervous system dominates our experience. When we activate the relaxation response, it is the parasympathetic that comes to the fore. This controls digestion, breathing, and heart rate during times when we are at rest, relaxing, using visualisations, meditating and sleeping. It is the parasympathetic nervous system that is concerned with the body's repair, maintenance and renewal.

In the relaxation response:

- heart rate is reduced, and the heart beats more effectively
- blood pressure is reduced
- blood is directed towards the internal organs, especially to those involved with digestion
- breathing rate is reduced as oxygen demand is reduced
- sweat production decreases
- digestion is improved through an increase in digestive enzyme secretions
- blood sugar levels remain constant.

There are many different types of relaxation techniques that elicit the relaxation response. These range from prayer and silent contemplation to meditation, progressive relaxation and breathing exercises. We all need to find our own best way to activate this healing for ourselves.

Relaxation Techniques

Consider joining a class to learn some relaxation skills. This gets you out of your usual environment and puts you in touch with new people, which in itself can help facilitate change in your life. Once learned and experienced, it will be easier for you to make the space for regular relaxation in your everyday routine. There are many different types of relaxation class, but they will all focus on one way of strengthening your body–mind link through three standard relaxation skills. These are:

- relaxing your body physically (eg clench your fist and then relax it to feel the difference)
- telling your body to relax with your mind or voice (eg imagine your body relaxing, or repeat some key words that will encourage you to let go)
- relaxing your mind (using guided imagery, meditation, etc).

Most techniques use a combination of all three. For all the relaxation exercises, follow these guidelines:

- choose somewhere that you will not be disturbed
- make yourself very comfortable, but try not to do them in bed because there is too much of a likelihood of you falling asleep
- allow yourself enough time to fully benefit from the exercise by taking an additional few minutes afterwards before getting back into everyday reality.

Progressive Relaxation

This uses a simple technique of comparing what it feels like to be tensed, to the pleasurable feelings of relaxation. It is a good exercise to start with because it is rich with information about how your body feels. You need to follow the previous guidelines for making both time and a comfortable space in which to do this exercise. You are going to work through your body, tensing specific muscles or muscle groups as tight as you can for a second or two, and then relaxing them. You will get to experience both the sensations of being relaxed and the process of relaxing in every part of your body, and the cumulative effect is a state of deep, full-body relaxation.

Start by contracting the muscles of your face and neck, hold for one to two seconds, and then relax them all. Follow this procedure with the muscles of your upper arms and chest, then your lower arms and hands. Work on down through your abdomen, buttocks, hips and thighs, calves and feet. When you get to the end of your body, return to your face and neck and repeat the whole body sweep two more times.

Once you are used to using this exercise and identifying different areas of your body, you may like to try using verbal cues instead of tensing and then relaxing each area in turn. For instance, consider starting the exercise with the spoken or silent: 'I am starting to experience full relaxation...My forehead, jaw, my whole face and neck are feeling comfortable, smooth and relaxed,' etc.

Muscular Relaxation

Follow the previous guidelines in preparation for this exercise. Close your eyes, and take a few deep, relaxed breaths, and feel your body start to relax a little. Notice the support you feel under your feet, your bottom, and your back, and enjoy the feelings of warmth and well-being that this engenders.

You are going to work your way through your body, relaxing each part of it by breathing out any tension that you find there. You can start at your head or toes, and work your way through your whole body to the other tip. With each breath become aware of the body part you are wanting to relax, and then breathe out from that place, releasing any tightness or disharmony and letting it be carried out of your body on your breath. Move on to the next spot and again breathe right into it before exhaling and letting go of any unwanteds. If you start at your left foot, move on to your left calf, your left shin, the knee, thigh and hip, before going on to the right foot. Stay in any area that you feel is extra tense, or not too responsive, continuing the flow of the breathing and your visualisations until you feel the area relax, and then carry on.

When you have covered your whole body, bring your attention to your breathing. Take a few deep, easy breaths down into the area of your belly button, and breathe right out from there. Take your time before slowly opening your eyes and stretching out your arms and legs. Stay still for a few minutes before getting on with your day.

Light Relaxation

Use your strong imaginative powers to connect your feelings of muscular relaxation with the image of a light bulb being switched off. As with the last exercise go through your body part by part, this time switching off the lights. You should begin to feel the warmth and softness that comes with increased relaxation. Use this as a night-time relaxer to prepare your body for sleep, and reverse it in the morning – skipping through your body and turning on all the lights to wake yourself up.

Another variation on this technique is to say to yourself as you relax each part of your body that it is becoming warm and heavy. Repeat 'My arm is becoming warm and heavy,' in your mind a few times, and wait until you notice this sensation in your arm before moving on to the next body part. Work your way through the body and when you are finished, move your attention to the forehead, and say to yourself 'My forehead feels cool.' Stay focused on your forehead for a moment or two and then say to yourself 'I feel refreshed and relaxed.'

Breathing Exercises

These have a special place in enhancing our relaxation response.

Simple, easy and relaxed breathing is a skill. It is something that we think we are doing all of the time, but most of us do not breathe in the most effective or relaxing way for most of the time. If you take a moment now to check your posture, you may find that your shoulders are raised a little too close to your ears, or that you are having to work those neck muscles to hold the weight of your head, or can identify a small knot of tension somewhere in your stomach or abdomen. These are all indicators of diaphragmatic tension, and they can all be reduced by breathing well.

The best breathing pattern is one that is deep and full, using the diaphragm to its best effect, and maintaining your own natural rhythm. The diaphragm is a strong muscle that sits right across your body and moves up and down in a rhythmic wave with every breath you take.

Relaxed Breathing

Sit comfortably and take a few deep breaths to settle yourself. Place one hand on your upper chest, just underneath your throat, and place your other on your stomach close to your belly button. Take another few breaths, and see which hand moves. Ideally, the hand covering your belly button should move in and out with each full, deep breath. Shallow breathing doesn't allow you to take in all the oxygen the body needs, nor does it let the lungs work properly and fully. You will know if your breathing is shallow because your upper hand will move up and down, magnifying the movement in the top of your chest.

Deep, relaxed breathing allows your diaphragm muscle to be exercised, and gives a gentle massage to all your internal organs with each new breath. It is a calming and supportive act that will form the basis for all the breathing techniques you use, as well as bringing calm into your daily life with each new breath you take.

You can learn to breathe more deeply by focusing your attention on the hand that is covering your belly button. Take each breath in right down as far as there, and breathe out from there too. Let your shoulders relax and loosen your waistband to encourage you. When you are breathing fully and deeply your upper hand will hardly move at all. Once you have experienced the difference, you will be able to return to this way of breathing whenever you think of it.

Breathe this way for at least five minutes every day, and you are likely to notice a number of positive side effects, such as improvement in the tone of your abdominal muscles, and feel a sense of deep relaxation. Once your body starts to appreciate the benefits this technique will feel more easy, and you will notice that you are taking deeper and smoother breaths quite naturally.

If you experience any lower back weakness this technique is not recommended for ongoing use because it can leave your lower back unsupported. In this situation it is better to practise breathing by widening your back and allowing your ribcage to expand within it, rather like a concertina. This will let you hold your lower abdominal muscles firm and taut, and protect the base of your spine. Here, again, the movement will not occur at the top of your chest, but rather at the back and sides of your ribcage.

Breathing with the Moon

This is a lovely technique that can be especially balancing for women. The moon has a deep connection with women and our changing monthly cycle and has been used as a symbol for this since ancient times. The moon goes through its own clear cycle each month, growing into fullness over 11 days, then holding its fullness for 3 days, before waning over 11 days and disappearing from view for about 4 days. We can find these four clear aspects within ourselves in the stages of our menstrual cycle, and in many of the things we undertake – all our projects follow the organic process of growing and having a point of fulfilment, as well as a time when their influence wanes and they become forgotten, or lost from sight. This exercise can reinforce our connection with our own cyclic nature and, if practised regularly, help regulate the menstrual cycle. (This can be extremely beneficial for enhancing fertility – practice mid-cycle when ovulation is due.) Alternatively, it can just be done after a spot of moon bathing for the magic and serenity it brings. I find it especially powerful to practise it with a full moon, and it is a good exercise to do on a retreat (see pp202–8).

Sit comfortably or lie down and relax – if possible within sight of the moon. Place the palm of the left hand over your belly button and the palm of your right lying over that. Take a few deep, easy breaths and settle yourself. Now, to a reasonably quick but steady count in your mind, breathe in to a count of 11, hold your breath for a slower count of 3, breathe out for another quick count of 11 and stay empty for a slower count of 4. Repeat the cycle as many times as you like.

Afterwards, you may like to open your eyes and gaze at the moon for a while to strengthen your sense of connection. This is a wonderful thing to do just before falling asleep, and you may find your dreams are touched by the exercise and your experience of it.

The Pelvic Breath

This is a wonderful exercise that combines deep relaxation with a deepening awareness of and sense of being really connected physically. It is good to do if you experience any period problems, because it may bring relief and insights as to how to remedy the situation further. It can also enhance the experience of a monthly retreat (see pp202–8).

Sit or lie down, and make yourself comfortable. Place your hands just below your belly button, and support your arms if necessary so that your hands can rest there comfortably. Close your eyes, and take a deep, cleansing breath. Now let each breath become a little deeper, and a little slower, until you feel that you are breathing right in down as far as your hands, and breathing out from that place too. The feeling should be slow, heavy, and relaxed. Imagine each breath carrying light into your pelvis, and illuminating the whole area, while you breathe out any disharmony or tension. Allow yourself to become fully involved in this process.

Continue breathing and let any images or ideas come into your mind about what your pelvis is like – might it be like a bowl that could contain things, or a garden in which things grow? Maybe it is something quite different – just see what comes to mind. Breathe in light with each new breath, and see what your pelvis holds as it is illuminated. Take your time, and stay with this exercise for as long as you like.

Finish by taking a few big, deep breaths, and moving your hands away from your pelvis. Stretch your body gently, as if you are waking up, and take another deep breath before opening your eyes.

You might like to write down your experience, or draw it or represent it in some way.

Meditation

Meditation is a profound experience that we can nevertheless access every moment of the day. It is a way of touching the very centre of our being, and remembering that connection in every part of us. It can give a sense of oneness with creation, or be a completely transcendent experience. When we meditate we learn about our own true nature, and have a chance to experience pure energy – the essence of ourselves. Being reminded of who we are in such a gentle, beautiful and peaceful way is truly life affirming. It enables us to move forwards in our lives in a more cohesive and purposeful way, and provides us with access to our own still centre whenever we need it.

Regular practise of meditation means we can reinforce the pathway to this still, calm and constant centre and build a strong memory-store of blissful feelings. It can infuse us with self-belief and steadiness in the most trying of times. It is a way through the sometimes chaotic life we lead into the arena of the sacred where we can feel the harmony of the universe, and experience ourselves vibrate in tune with it. Once you have experienced meditation, you will be able to approach anything that you do in a meditative way – whether it is preparing your meal or travelling to work.

There are many different techniques for achieving this stillness, and you may find some more appropriate than others – experience them for yourself and see. You can focus on using a mental image which you can concentrate on to the exclusion of all else, or follow sound to guide you through your maze of thoughts and feelings, or the movement of your breathing. The mechanics of all are much the same.

You will need to make some time for yourself when you will not be disturbed, and get into a comfortable position. This might be kneeling on the floor with a cushion for support, sitting cross-legged, or on a chair with your feet flat on the floor. Choose a position that keeps your spine straight. Take some time to get this right so you will not be distracted when you are sitting. Let your shoulders relax and your arms hang comfortably. Settle your hands in your lap or on your thighs, apart or cradled one in the other. Laying them palm side up is relaxing and signifies an openness about you. Set aside about 20 minutes when you first start, although you may find that you like to spend much longer in this state, or that shorter visits suit you more. Plan to meditate at the same time each day to introduce it as a regular pattern in your life.

When you are sitting, endeavour to stay quite still, although you may find yourself making some involuntary movements as your energy shifts and postural muscles are able to relax.

Awareness Meditation

Close your eyes and become aware of what is around you – the support underneath your bottom; the touch of the air on your skin; the sounds you can hear from outside. Visit all these things with your attention so that you are aware of everything that is happening around you. Now bring your awareness to your upper lip, and the feelings and sensations of your breath. Don't stress about your breathing pattern, just notice the area in the middle of your top lip where you feel your breath. Hold your concentration there without forcing it – explore the area and the sensations you feel. Notice all the changes from temperature to pressure. If you find yourself being distracted, gently draw your attention back to this place.

Part of the exercise is to be able to draw yourself back from the seductive pull of other thoughts to this simple spot where you can directly experience one of the most amazing aspects of your life – your breath. When you are content to sit and focus on the point where you feel your breath come and go, you can move on with it – be aware of yourself breathing in and breathing out. Notice, but don't judge or try to change, the flow and your own unique rhythm. Be aware of whatever part of yourself you feel to be 'doing' the breathing and stay there for a while to explore this.

Then you may become aware of the breath itself. It is inside your body, but it is still the air that is outside of your body touching your skin. That is part of the air that surrounds your entire body, and fills the room you are in. Breathing means you create your own tidal flow that affects all the air around you. Continue breathing in and out at your own pace and hold your attention on the breath. This may take a few times to relax into, because you need to experience it, rather than thinking your way through it. Once you are able to let go of the thoughts and directions you are likely to experience something quite amazing that will raise questions, and provide answers all at the same time, but the art of meditation is to stay with the experience rather than being caught by the appeal of solving the mystery, and the only way to do this is to try it for yourself.

You will know when it is time to stop – sometimes because your body will not be able to stay still any more, or because your mind will become too demanding. This will change with practice and over time. When you are ready, slowly bring your awareness back to the point on your lip where you can feel your breathing, and from there to the rest of your body – once more feeling the support underneath your bottom and the feel of air all over your skin.

Take a few minutes to get yourself back into ordinary, everyday reality. Take a few deep, easy breaths, and have a gentle stretch. Open your eyes carefully, and do not touch your face or head for a few minutes.

Guided Imagery

This is a wonderful way to relax. It involves using your powerful imagination and will involve your body in a quite amazing way. When you believe something to be true, your body will respond as though it is, so if you can create a strong enough image of yourself lying on a sun-kissed desert island beach, you will be able to truly experience all the benefits.

We use this skill all the time when we daydream or wish for things, and formalising it like this with a structure and revisiting it often makes a truly beneficial skill from something we often take for granted. You can experience this for yourself right now by returning in your mind's eye to a favourite real or fantasy location, and imagining yourself to be there. Notice how safe and secure you feel in your own energy, and how relaxed you are, and how pleasurable it is. The best thing of all about this is that you don't need any equipment, or tools, just the desire to do it. You can practise this whenever and wherever you choose.

At its simplest, you can use your imagination to help with your stress levels by simply breathing out any tension that you notice in your body, and imagining the stress and tightness leaving your body on the breath. Use pictures in your mind to reinforce the effect. For instance:

- ice melting to dissipate the stress
- the sun's rays reaching down and warming you to loosen up the area
- breathing out muddy colours or greyness and breathing in pure, white light or a rainbow
- untying or undoing knots in muscles that might look like ropes or twisted ribbons.

Or you may find that you spontaneously receive your own helpful and healing images that will be personal to you.

On a larger scale, you can return in your mind's eye to a favourite real or fantasy location, and imagine yourself there. Building this skill will enhance your relaxation response and increase your body's ability to relax on cue. Experience the two following scenarios for yourself to see how much detail and richness you can incorporate into your imaginings, and then spend some time regularly enjoying this aspect of your life.

You can read these suggestions onto a tape, or have them read to you to maximise the relaxational benefit. Leave long gaps between sentences to allow your own images to develop and let you savour the experience fully. Working slowly enables you to build up the layers of images in your mind and will greatly enhance the experience. Choose somewhere comfortable where you will not be disturbed, close your eyes and prepare to relax and enjoy...

Visiting the Seaside
See yourself walking barefoot along the seashore.
Feel the warm sand between your toes.
Listen to the sound of the waves gently 'shooshing' on to the shore.
See the magnificent scenery that surrounds you and appreciate the full palette of colours.

Become aware of the warmth on your skin, and the calls of the seabirds as they fly nearby.
Notice yourself smile as a coconut falls out of a tree and rolls towards you.
Smell and taste the salt carried on the warm air.

Just ahead of you, notice a small pool of fresh water.
As you get closer to it, see how the sunlight glints gently on the polished surface of the water, and lets you see below some of the beautiful shells that are resting there.
Settle yourself by the pool and let yourself take a deep breath in and enjoy the experience.

A Woodland Scene

See yourself walking slowly along a woody path.
Feel the gentle touch of new leaves brushing against your skin and the dappled sunlight teasing your senses as it peeks between the trees.
Listen to the rushing sound of water cascading down into a nearby pool, and smell the heady scents of jasmine and rose being wafted along on a light refreshing breeze.
Watch as the dragonflies dance beautifully over the path ahead of you and hear the frogs chirruping, and the occasional cry of a bird passing overhead.
Hear the gentle 'swash' as the treetops sway in the breeze.
Enjoy the slightly musky smell of being in a wood.

As you reach the waterfall, sit down on the edge of the pool and marvel at the clear water, and the refreshing sensations as you dangle your feet in it.

Take a sip of the cool, cleansing water, and enjoy the heavy sensation as it drips through your fingers and back into the pool

Lean forward slightly, and gaze for a while at your own reflection, then lie down and let your body relax into the support of the woodland floor while you continue to enjoy the sounds and scents that surround you.

Using an Anchor

This is a simple little technique that is profoundly effective in reminding you of the way you felt when you were supremely relaxed, totally capable, happy and fully in control. You can develop an anchor of your choice using any of the relaxation exercises or techniques that you practise. Then when you are feeling anxious or stress is mounting, using your anchor will remind your body of this other way of feeling. It is very effective.

You can choose a physical anchor such as touching your wrist with your other hand, or placing both hands palm down at your side. Or you can choose a verbal or mental anchor – a phrase which you repeat to yourself, such as 'I am safe and secure in my own energy' or 'I feel calm, relaxed and in control.' The best of these anchors are just one word that holds a lot of meaning for you, and that you are unlikely to forget.

When you have decided upon your anchor, plan to introduce it the next time you do a relaxation technique. When you reach a point where you are fully relaxed, and are simply enjoying the feelings and sensations of being in this supremely carefree state, then either repeat to yourself silently your word or phrase, or move your body in the required way. Be clear in your mind that you are going to remember this phrase, word, posture or movement as a short cut to remembering these good feelings. Repeat this introduction at each peak relaxation point over the next week or so to strengthen your connection and increase its effectiveness. You can continue to reinforce it every time you relax if you like, but it is the first week or so that is really needed to learn it properly. Then when you feel yourself becoming stressed, you can take a moment and use your anchor. It will remind you of the good feelings and awaken your body's memory, and will change your experience of the situation you are in.

Relaxing Your Life

The regular use of relaxation techniques will have a positive effect on your ability to deal with stressful situations, and will work to lower your level of arousal. Beyond these specific exercises there are many different types of things that we find good sources of relaxation, and it is essential that we embrace a more balanced approach to our lives and prioritise relaxing experiences into our daily schedule.

The following chapters look at a range of different ways to induce and enhance the relaxation response, starting with the role of food in our ability to relax.

Chapter 4 – Food

A good diet is essential to managing stress and to promoting harmony in our lives. The foods we eat provide us with regular and reliable sources of energy, and making good food choices means we do not create internal stress. Our diet is the source of all our renewable hormones, and our only way to replenish stores of protein building blocks and other essential material. When and how we eat, as well as our choice of food, will impact upon the body's internal stress levels. Food can act as our most immediate medicine when we use it wisely, gently restoring digestion after the effects of long-term stress, and providing a host of medicinal benefits.

Some food elements are of special interest to us in maintaining equilibrium in the face of stress. For instance, high potassium/low sodium foods need to be in abundance in the diet to ensure we can counteract the effects of aldosterone in maintaining high blood pressure. We need to watch the type of fats we eat in order to not put an even greater burden on the heart (see pp101–2), as well as to supply the building materials for some of our hormonal needs. Proteins need careful handling too in order to meet our requirements in a non-stressful way. Specific foods and types of foods will also have a stress-busting effect in terms of reinforcing our nervous system: B complex vitamins are essential to strong neural function and development; vitamin C is essential to promote repair and strengthen our immune response, and the comfort and calcium in a range of warming foods such as milky drinks and sweet halva are effective at calming any feelings of jitteriness and tension.

The benefits of a good everyday diet are long-term. Making sure we have a good resource of all the nutrients we need means we are less likely to suffer the stress of nutritional deficiencies. Any individual food allergies or sensitivities, the presence of chemicals and preservatives in our diet along with an array of waxes, colourants, flavourisers, etc, and the preparation and storage methods we employ all impact upon the delivery of the optimum nutrition which we need to function at our best.

Food can be an emotive subject for many of us who are not encouraged to nurture ourselves. It is also a very clear area where we can exercise control over our lives, and is involved in many addictive patterns. Also, our attitude towards food, and towards ourselves, can alter during the changing hormonal patterns of our monthly cycle.

One of the most important things about food, and the way to maximise its numerous benefits, is to enjoy it. For many of us, relaxing and savouring the deliciousness and the positive nature of foods is a very difficult task. We are conditioned into believing that this essential substance is something we need to manipulate in order to maintain our weight and good figure. We are repeatedly sold the lie that the best food choices we can make for ourselves are those that contain no calories, and therefore no nourishment at all, so we can tend to rely on ready-made foods and snacks which contain very little nutrition. A recent study showed that most single women under 30 years old spend only half an hour per day on preparing and eating meals, but over two hours per day watching television.

Revisiting the pleasure and power of being in charge of your own positive nourishment is a lifesaving act. Every time you eat something because it is a good health choice, you make an amazingly positive two-fold statement. You give your body something it will benefit from and reinforce your health. You also release yourself from the stress of counting calories or choosing foods that are included in whatever slimming diet you happen to be currently following. Every time you choose good food and opt to savour the delights or the sensual pleasures of a meal, you reinforce your own sense of deserving the very best. Each act of pleasure is a positive rebellion against the system that seeks to remove your power, whether you see this as the pressures of society or some more personal demons.

A Good Basic Diet

The definition of what constitutes a good basic diet will change according to a number of factors. Energy needs change according to what we are doing. For instance, growing children and pregnant women require a lot more protein, calcium and other vitamins and minerals than at any other time, and having a period can increase pure energy needs for the fuel we get from carbohydrates by up to 50 per cent. Over the course of each monthly cycle we can introduce days when we naturally fast or eat a light diet and days when we can feast. This means that we can have days when we rest the digestive system and days when we can relax our own dietary rules. Feast days are especially good around the time of our period, when we need an increased calorie intake and usually benefit from some degree of personal indulgence.

Nutrition from food comes in different forms so we need to choose a variety of foods to make sure we get the vitamins, minerals, trace elements, protein, fats, carbohydrates and fibre that we need each day. Many foods contain several types of energy (eg grains contain carbohydrate, minerals and fibre) and this will change according to how it is stored, prepared and cooked. Foods are mainly classified by their major constituent.

Protein

Protein needs vary enormously between individuals and through the course of our lives. We need about 10 per cent of our total calorie intake to be protein, and we need some protein every day because the body does not make its own and does not store any excess. Its work in the body is to provide the energy and the building blocks for new growth and repair. Protein sources are one of the more controversial issues about our diet. If you choose to include animal protein in your diet, you must choose the freshest and best quality. It is essential that the animals are organically and well reared, or wild and humanely slaughtered. Otherwise the build-up of toxins, antibiotics and other drugs, hormones, nitrates and other chemicals in the system is too great for the food to be of any real benefit to us. And of course there are also moral issues to consider. Nuts, seeds, beans, pulses, peas and grains are all good sources of protein, and it is also present in cheese, eggs and milk.

Sprouting grains and seeds is an excellent way to source protein, vitamins and minerals. Sprout mung beans, aduki beans, sunflower seeds and anything else you fancy quickly and easily in a glass jar on your draining board. Pour on and then drain a little warm water. Refresh the beans this way three or four times a day. They will sprout within two to six days, and be both nutritious and delicious.

Carbohydrates

Carbohydrates are our main source of energy, and come from a wide range of sources. They also provide protein, vitamins and minerals. The bulk of our diet, about 60 per cent, should be made up of unrefined carbohydrates. They include the starches such as those in bread; sugars like those in milk and fruit; and the fibre we get from vegetables, pulses, seeds and nuts. Good carbohydrates include cereals, seeds, roots and tubers, eg rice, corn, pasta, bulgur, couscous, rye, buckwheat, parsnips, celeriac, carrots and beetroot.

Fats

Fats are necessary for a range of activities including the production of some hormones (see p19), the absorption of fat-soluble vitamins, and for insulation. Fats also provide energy. They need to make up only a small part of our diet in order to fulfil our daily needs, and less than 30 per cent is a good figure to aim for. Eating them early in a meal is most useful. Saturated fats mainly come from animals, and although they provide a very concentrated form of energy, we need to minimise them because of their connection with cardiovascular disease and their lack of the additional benefits which other types of fat provide. Monounsaturated fats come from nuts, seeds and olives and are good substitutes for saturated fats. Polyunsaturated fats are involved in making the adrenal and sex hormones as well as maintaining a healthy population of bacteria in the gut. These are readily available as fish and fish oils, nuts and nut oils, and vegetable oils. They also contain EFAs (essential fatty acids) which are vital for a healthy immune system and a healthy nervous system. Together with proteins, EFAs form the major structural part of the cell wall in every cell in the body.

Fibre

Increased fibre and water helps peristalsis (the way food is moved through the gut), and keeps things moving. Fibre is found in the skin and cell walls of fruits and vegetables – so we receive more when we can eat them unpeeled and raw or very lightly cooked. You can only really eat the skins of fruit and vegetables that have been naturally or organically grown. Fibre is also found in seeds, pulses, beans and grains that have not been refined and stripped of their outer, fibre-rich layers.

Vitamins and Minerals

Vitamins and minerals are a wide range of essential nutrients that effect myriad different positive health activities within the body. They are often considered as supplements, but are present in almost all of the food we eat provided they have not been destroyed or stripped away. The full range of these vitamins and minerals is essential to full health. Vitamins are divided into those which are soluble in water like the B-complex, and C, and those which require fat to be absorbed, such as A and E. Much of the vitamin and mineral content of food will depend upon the condition of the soil in which it was grown (inland soil tends to be iodine deficient, and the levels of selenium in soil vary widely) and the way it is then stored and prepared.

Storage is important because the longer a food is kept, the less vitamins it is likely to have left. They start to die off once a vegetable or fruit is picked, and are killed by exposure to air, light and heat. Growing your own, even if it is just a few lettuce plants in a window box, or some cress and parsley in pots in the kitchen, is the best way to ensure you have a mega-dose of vitamins each day. Preparing food requires some care to make sure you make the most of what you have. Always wash food before you cut or chop it, and prepare it as close to cooking time as possible.

Cooking destroys many of the vitamins in fruit and vegetables, but makes the food softer, warmer and easier to digest. When you boil vegetables in water and then throw the water down the sink, you are throwing away most of the goodness. Make the most of your cooking methods by using the cooking water as a base for soups, gravy, etc, or cook in a steamer.

Vitamins and Minerals

Vitamin	Found in:	Destroyed by:
A	Fish oils, milk produce, egg yolk, carrots, precursor carotene in all yellow and orange veg and fruits, dandelion leaves, parsley and watercress	Heat (with air) and some metals
B complex	see p126	Heat, air, light, and water
C	Fresh fruit and vegetables, leafy herbs, berries	Heat, air, water, alkalinity and some enzymes and metals
D	Milk and milk products, eggs, fish and fish oils and produced by action of sun on your skin	Air, heat
E	Nuts, seeds, whole grains, seaweeds, soy beans	Air, heat
K	Green vegetables, milk, molasses, apricots, sunflower oil. Synthesised in the gut.	Harmful bacteria

Mineral		
Sodium	Most vegetables, salt, seaweeds	All minerals can be leached by water
Calcium	see pp123–5	These are all specifically indicated in the treatment of stress and are covered in more detail later in this chapter
Iron	see pp125–6	
Magnesium	see p122	
Potassium	see p122	
Phosphorus	Whole grains, weeds, nuts fish	
Copper	Green vegetables, seafoods, whole grains	

Zinc	Oysters, herrings, yeast, eggs, peas, seeds, fruit, vegetables, nuts
Cobalt	Brewer's yeast, fruit, vegetables, whole grains, nuts
Manganese	Green vegetables, seeds, whole grains and pulses
Iodine	Seaweeds and seafoods, parsley, iodised salt, vegetables grown near the sea
Chromium	Fruit, vegetables, molasses, whole grains, wheatgerm, organically grown produce
Selenium	Garlic, whole grains, brewer's yeast, produce from selenium-rich soil.

Supplements

Ideally, most of the nutrients we need should come from the food we eat, but this is not possible when we make extra demands on our body, and when the quality of the food we eat has been compromised in some way – perhaps by being chemically grown, or as a mass produced 'fast food'. Supplementation is then an effective answer to ensure that our short-term needs are met.

Taking an all-round supplement is a good way to ensure extra support for your body at times when you most need it. Take your tablet or capsule with a meal, ideally with your last few mouthfuls, or with a drink immediately afterwards. Some nutrients are compromised or destroyed by heat, so choose a small glass of water or juice.

There are many types of multivitamin and mineral products available, and this is an area where you need to be every bit as vigilant as you are with your food choices. It is not desirable to choose a product that contains artificial sweeteners, colourings, preservatives, etc. These will not benefit your health, and can add their weight to the internal stress your body experiences. Make sure that the product you choose is free from all additives, and if possible select one that is yeast, dairy and sugar free. You will also need to ensure that the vitamins are in a natural form that is easily accessible to your body.

Some vitamins and minerals are specially involved in the maintenance of good nerves, strong digestion, and a positive immune response. These are all key factors in managing stress. These can have positive benefits when they are used to enhance everyday diet, and focus on areas most in need of support. It is not necessary to take these separately, but look for adequate levels of them in your multiple formula.

Key vitamins and minerals and the optimum levels to look for in supplements include:

- vitamin B complex – levels will vary for individual vitamins
- vitamin C – 500 mg, although it may be easier to take in smaller doses of 250 mg. Look too for

accompanying bioflavonoids to aid absorption. This is one vitamin that you can take in addition to your multi (see further information below)

- vitamin E – 30 IU
- calcium – 700 mg
- magnesium – 400 mg
- iron – around 9 mg but variable according to form. We lose 15–30 mg with each period, but this is a difficult mineral to supplement with successfully. (It can cause constipation and not be absorbed by the body.) Best choice is separate supplementation with iron of vegetable origin in a liquid form, such as Floradix or Floravital
- zinc – 15 mg. This is not suitable for long-term use. Take for two to three months only, then rest for at least one month
- manganese – 2 mg. This is especially important because long-term deficit can easily occur
- selenium – 150 mcg
- chromium – 25 µg.

Stress-busting Supplements

If you are under a lot of stress, consider taking the following supplements to support your body. Do not take them for more than one month in four. If you feel you need specific advice that is right for your body and your lifestyle, then see a natural healthcare practitioner.

- Vitamin C – take up to 3 g a day for short periods of time. You will know when your body has had enough because you will develop diarrhoea. Reduce the dose until your bowel movements return to normal, and keep it as high as your body will tolerate. This is best taken in small, frequent doses, so look for a 250 mg or 500 mg product, or choose a vitamin C powder that you can measure into drinks.

- B complex – take a balanced formula at the dose recommended. Do not supplement with individual B vitamins without your practitioner's advice, because this can throw you further off balance.
- Pycnogenol – a fantastic antioxidant that will benefit your entire system and reinforce the work of vitamin C. This is a wonderful energiser. Take as directed.
- Echinacea – either as tincture or tablet. Take this for 10 days, then give yourself a three- to five-day break. This will stimulate your immune system and strengthen your body.
- Ginseng – a tonic which increases energy levels and supports the adrenal glands. Take daily as a standardised extract in capsules or tablets, taking 20 mg of the active ingredient.
- Acidophilus – this is available in tablet, capsule or powder form and will enhance effective digestion by increasing the levels of beneficial bacteria in your gut. It is advisable to take a course of this after any antibiotic treatment, or when you experience thrush or other fungal complaints. It is also good to stabilise digestion after long-term stress. Always store your acidophilus in the fridge because heat destroys it, and take with a cold drink away from meals.

Assessing Your Diet

Although supplements need to be taken every day, it may be useful to balance your food intake by the week, rather than on a daily basis. This way you can tailor your diet towards the end of the week to make up any shortfalls from the beginning, and this also allows for more flexibility while you are developing your skill and knowledge in this area.

The fresher the foods you eat, and the more varied your diet, the more likely you are to be providing yourself with the full range of nutrients that you need. Make sure that you have some raw food every day. Choosing a selection of seasonal vegetables and dressing them simply with some olive oil and freshly squeezed lime or lemon juice will maximise the energy you get from your meal and make sure you get some extra vitamin C.

Try to include the following in your diet each day:

- fresh, raw fruit and vegetables
- fresh fruit or vegetable juice
- cooked fruit and vegetables
- grains, eg wheat, rice, rye, corn, buckwheat, barley
- nuts, seeds, pulses
- protein.

Keeping a Diet Diary

Record what you eat through the week in a daily diet diary. This is often used to identify any possible allergens or food sensitivity, but it is also good for providing a clear look at how balanced your everyday food intake is. Keep a diary every day for a week and write in it everything that you eat and drink, when you have it (this is very important), and also make a note of how you are feeling. Your daily page could look something like this:

Day and date:	Time:	Feelings:
Breakfast		
Drinks		
Lunch		
Drinks		
Snacks		
Drinks		
Dinner		
Drinks		

At the end of each day you can review the overall balance of your diet and make plans for the next day's food. This will also highlight any over-dependence you may have on one particular food or food group. Wheat and dairy foods, for instance, are the most common causes of health concerns being implicated in a range of complaints from arthritis to eczema and sinusitis. They are both mucus producing and can cause lazy digestion, but they are both likely to appear frequently in the diet – often as toast or a wheat-based breakfast cereal covered with milk, then as a sandwich for lunch – possibly cheese? – and as pasta with parmesan for dinner. If you notice any foods appearing often on your daily sheets you may like to consider alternatives for them to widen your dietary intake and reduce the associated health challenges. Look to the substitution table at the end of this chapter, or consider consulting a naturopath or natural healthcare practitioner for a personalised assessment of your dietary needs.

Home-cooked foods are almost always better, if only because they are likely to be fresher, and may be more lovingly prepared, than anything you can buy. Eating out may also mean eating more foods that are high in fat and salt. Check your diet diary for potential hidden extras from meals eaten out, and endeavour to have at least one home-cooked meal each day.

When assessing your diet you will also want to take into account the season, and your own health concerns.

The Energy of Food

The energetic quality of food is as important as its classification as a protein, carbohydrate or fat. Some foods work specifically to enhance different areas of our body – eg yellow foods, containing vitamin A, such as carrots, corn and squash are helpful to the spleen and its work of producing new blood cells. These are good foods to eat when balancing the menstrual cycle.

Foods that are heating and over-stimulating may exacerbate our sense of being stressed, when cooler, more calming foods would be a better remedy.

Including gently warming spices and herbs to encourage digestion can help us recover after the long-term effects of stress have been to close down our digestive system.

Warming foods include fish and meat and all animal products, especially egg yolks, and obviously heating foods such as chillies. Less obvious are carrots, berries, citrus fruits, beetroot, fenugreek, garlic, mustard, salt (see pp114–15), cumin, horseradish, onions, peppers, radish, sesame seeds, alcohol and tomatoes. Corn and wheat are two of the most warming grains. Sugar is intensely heating (see pp113–14) and other warming sweeteners include honey and molasses.

When used in moderation, these foods can warm digestion and stimulate the appetite, in excess they can aggravate and overstimulate the nervous system. They need to be used carefully in the presence of stress-related concerns, when the worst over-stimulation comes from garlic, alcohol, mustard, chilli and fish.

Cooling foods tend to calm us down and can be especially useful during the warmer months and when stress-related agitation is high. In excess, they can make digestion slow and heavy, so use in balance with the heating foods above, and more neutral foods such as sweet fruits, basmati rice and mung beans.

The most cooling foods are coriander leaf and seed, black raisins (preferably soaked and partially rehydrated) celery, courgette, peas, aduki beans, soya beans and their products (but not soya sauce which tends to be heating, as are all fermented foods), coconut, cottage cheese, egg whites, saffron, fennel, anise, mint, lemon balm and rose.

Caffeine

Caffeine can over-stimulate and add enormously to feelings of being stressed and under pressure. It stimulates the nervous system, making it overactive, and will interfere with good sleep. It also increases the heart rate, and can cause irregularities in the beat. It will add to indigestion and other digestive concerns that are stress-related, and can increase blood cholesterol levels to higher than optimum levels. Reducing your caffeine intake is one of the best changes you can make to calm and re-balance your body.

Caffeine contents vary according to how strong you take your coffee (filter coffee contains approximately 240 mg per cup, percolated coffee 192 mg, and instant 104 mg), and what brand you use, but more than 750 mg a day is not desirable, and the lower your levels, the calmer you will feel. Never take caffeine after 4 pm or it will impact upon your getting to sleep. Caffeine is also present in tea (a cup of brewed tea contains 75 mg), cola drinks (around 300 mg in a small can), and chocolate (a mug of cocoa contains about 300 mg and a small bar of plain chocolate has close to 250 mg).

Sugar

Sugar is present in most of the foods we eat, but it is usually contained within cells that take some time and effort for the body to access – so we have to work for it. This is a very good thing. It is often also present alongside a range of other nutrients, vitamins and minerals that all benefit the body. Refined sugar is like a poison that blasts energy levels through the roof without giving any nutrients, or having any of the buffers that food generally contains. It can be a great aid when facing severe physical challenges that require you to respond immediately, or when your personal resources are too low to react normally. Otherwise, it just sets up an imbalance that will see you reeling from energy peaks to periods of deep slump and tiredness, when the temptation of a quick energy 'fix' will be even greater.

We can all manage quite effectively without adding any additional sugar to our diets, and if you give yourself some time to experience this, you will soon get to enjoy the smoother, more relaxed feeling of constant energy, without the rushes and lows that sugar produces. If you must add sugar, take it in very small amounts, and in a form that at least brings some benefits with it – honey, raw cane sugar that is filled with minerals, and maple syrup are possible alternatives.

Salt

Salt adds to the flavour of food, but in too great a quantity it can swamp the taste, and it is implicated in a range of health concerns. There is a definite link with raised blood pressure, and we need to ensure high potassium levels in the diet to manage stress effectively. These are unbalanced in the presence of sodium. (See pp133–4.) Processed foods contain much more salt than unprocessed, and plant foods contain much less than animal-based foods. Reducing your salt levels will calm and settle you, allow your taste buds to reawaken to the natural flavours in your food, and should help keep blood pressure more stable. Bacon is an obvious example of a salty food, and it contains about 81 mcg sodium per 100 g. Salted butter contains 38, tomato ketchup 49, lettuce 0.4, potatoes 0.3 and apples 0.1.

When, How and Where We Eat

These factors can be as important as what you actually choose to eat. Simply making time to eat and enjoy your meal in a settled environment will reduce your stress levels in two very important ways – by making for a real break from your other activities, and by ensuring that you maximise your digestive ability. Your system is designed to benefit most from regular meals, and we have already seen how we need to be relaxed in order to digest and assimilate the food we eat. Making sure you keep to regular mealtimes will enable your body to relax into the sure knowledge that more energy will be coming soon. It lets your body budget, and gives it something to rely on, as well as providing fresh resources at regular intervals. Eating regularly also cuts down on the amount of adrenaline you have in your system. Digestion begins in your mouth, and chewing food thoroughly increases your sense of satisfaction and feelings of fullness, enhances its flavour, and ensures thorough and efficient digestion.

Endeavour to leave about four hours between meals or snacks to ensure a regular supply of energy throughout your day. When you have the physical energy to meet all your needs, you eliminate the stress that comes with the fear of not coping.

A good breakfast is an important start to the day, and whatever you eat and drink first thing in the morning will fire up your system and prepare you for the day ahead. It replenishes you after what may be a twelve-hour or even longer fast, and warms your digestion ready for the day's work. We each have our own capacity for this meal, but it is good to eat something. Experiment for a week with a range of different menu choices to see what type of meal you respond to best at this time of the day. Choose: fresh sour fruit such as grapefruit or strawberries and toast; or warmed up leftovers from the previous night (to see if you prefer a savoury meal); or scrambled eggs or spicy scrambled tofu with rice or on toast; or porridge with soya 'milk' and honey; or pancakes or waffles with stewed berries or apple; or sweet fruit like apple, banana, mango or papaya with warm, spiced fruit juice or herbal tea; or bagels or a muffin with a cup of decaffeinated coffee or hot chocolate made with soya 'milk'; or whole-grain cereal with soya 'milk'; kedgeree or warmed fish; or meusli with hot apple juice and added fruit. Make a note of your energy levels through the morning, and your appetite for lunch, as well as how you feel after eating.

Digestion is usually at its peak around noon, and food eaten then is processed and assimilated more easily and completely. This means maximum nutritional benefit for the least energy output – a good internal equation. Nowadays, we seem to have less and less time for food preparation and for meals. Squeezing a lunch break seems like one of the easiest ways to make more time in the day, but nearly one third of working women don't take a lunch break at all, and less than half routinely make time for this essential meal, even to eat a sandwich at their desk! Many of us take a packed lunch to work, and this is an easy and inexpensive way to make sure that we get the nourishment we need in the form we want, but it is essential to make the time for it.

Do not eat less than two hours before going to bed so that you can digest and assimilate the meal, rather than leaving it undigested in your stomach over night. Even though you spend much of your night asleep, your body is still working and it is important that you give yourself some more fuel when you wake up in the morning.

Snacks

Snacks are an important part of all our days, and this is especially true in the few days each month when a period is due. Calorie needs rise at this time by up to 50 per cent, and eating something every two hours will do a lot to stave off some of the symptoms of PMS. Choose to snack on foods that will give you good energy, rather than the quick fix of sugar. Carbohydrates, whole-grain foods, grains, nuts, seeds, fruits and vegetables are all good choices. Snacks can be a useful way of maintaining energy levels when there is insufficient time in the schedule for regular mealtimes. Choose to have a number of snacks throughout the day if you are dealing with erratic energy levels, and seeking to boost your blood sugar levels.

A knowledge of food values means you will be able to make healthy choices to fit your own immediate needs. Some foods are of special interest to us because they can help balance our specific health needs, and these are discussed below. For snacks, yoghurt is calming to the digestion, and it can be sweetened with fresh fruit, and warmed with a pinch of cinnamon or turmeric to enhance digestion further. Add a teaspoon of honey to make an instant energy-booster. Dried apricots are an excellent aid to digestion, speeding peristalsis and removing any blockages, and will give a fast and easily used fix of energy. (But remember when eating only dried food that you will need to drink extra water too!) Raisins will help the body detox, and have a restorative and regenerative effect upon the system. They also provide instant energy. Peanuts are nutritious. They are high in B vitamins, and vitamin E, iron, protein and zinc. Other snack suggestions include:

- dried fruits
- nuts
- seeds
- oatcakes, rice cakes, corn cakes, etc
- popcorn
- Ryvita and other crispbreads
- fresh fruit
- mixed grain toasted cereals and mueslis
- freshly extracted juice (whisk in some live yoghurt for extra energy).

Be responsive to your own changing needs, and eat more frequently – perhaps several smaller meals – throughout the day if this is what suits you best.

The way you eat is also important. It is very good practice to sit down and make time for your meals, even if you are just snacking. Move away from your desk, or lay a place for yourself at the table, and structure the time as one for you to enjoy your own nourishment. Don't be tempted to work while you eat, and avoid discussing business, or scheduling regular business meetings for mealtimes. Seek out peaceful, harmonious surroundings that will enhance and benefit your experience – it can almost be more stressful to sit in a brightly lit, loud, bustling area while you eat than to skip a meal altogether.

Not Eating

Not eating occasionally is a good way to rest your digestive system, and you might consider eating very simply – perhaps only fruit, and drinking lots of water on one day each month. Choose to do this mid-cycle, when you are ovulating, for maximum benefits and increased ease when your period comes. Following some form of detox like this every month will encourage good digestion and relieve some of the dietary stress your body can experience.

Not eating is a natural response to illness, and your appetite may disappear when you are developing a cold or flu. When this happens, don't force yourself to eat, take lots of drinks, juices, teas and clear soup. Children often don't eat for a day at a time and this is nothing to worry about. It is a natural thing. If it happens regularly you might have them checked, and look to other worries that could be affecting them. Get rid of any tensions around eating and introduce some rules about no shouting, not having the TV on while you are sitting down together to eat, etc. Involve your child in the kitchen, and in food preparation and choices. Often 'picky' eaters will engage more if they have a part to play in mealtimes. If your child doesn't eat for more than twenty-four hours, and if they have any other symptoms of ill health, seek professional advice.

Food as Medicine

Some foods are of specific interest to us for their wide range of nutritional and healing properties.

Reducing Stress

Beyond a good basic diet, there is much that food can do to specifically reduce the ill effects of stress.

Keep your mealtimes as free from stress as possible by:

- eating regularly. Your body will relax if it knows it will receive the energy it needs at regular intervals through the day
- learning to recognise your hunger
- making sure you are comfortable – sit down to eat and seek an atmosphere that is relaxing and without disturbance
- attend to what you are doing – focus on your own positive nutrition rather than the bad news on TV, etc
- choose cooling foods if you or your digestion are agitated
- attend to key nutrient levels, specifically potassium, magnesium, calcium, iron and vitamins C and B complex
- reduce the amount of saturated fat in your diet, and increase the amount of fibre you eat.

Potassium

Maintaining potassium levels is key to managing stress. Aim to have 3–5 grams each day of potassium, and avoid sodium as much as possible. Do not add salt to your meals at the table – keep a good quality sea salt in the kitchen for cooking, and allow the flavour of the foods to develop, or enhance them with herbs and spices. Foods high in potassium (and low in sodium) are shown in the following table:

Food	Potassium	Sodium
(raw unless stated)		
1 medium apple	182 milligrams	2 milligrams
60 g dried apricots	318	9
1 medium banana	440	1
1 medium peach	308	2
5 strawberries	122	trace
small bunch of asparagus	165	1
½ avocado	680	5
1 medium-sized carrot	225	38
1 medium cooked potato	782	6
1 medium tomato	444	5
90 g cooked cod	345	93
90 g cooked haddock	297	150
90 g tinned tuna (drained)	225	38

Magnesium

Magnesium is an essential element that will ensure smooth muscle action and relieve period pains. It has myriad other functions in the body, and deficiency is very common. Find it in:

- watercress
- spinach
- raspberries
- parsley
- oats
- kelp
- dandelion
- figs and dates
- nuts
- seafood.

Calcium

Calcium needs also rocket during stress. This is an important element for us because of the risk of osteoporosis when bone density can be lost when we age. The presence of noradrenaline in the system on a long-term basis increases the excretion of calcium, so it needs to be taken daily. Calcium needs other elements such as boron and vitamins C and D to be used effectively in the body.

Calcium has been looked at in detail as an important element in balancing the effects of stress. It acts as a stomach buffer, and is involved in a complex balancing act with sodium and potassium to regulate a number of cellular activities, including the way muscles work. Calcium is also the primary element involved in the density of our bones. The loss of this is osteoporosis.

Sesame seeds are a wonderfully rich source of calcium and are essential for maintaining bone density and protecting against osteoporosis. Eat them on their own, added to a mix of other seeds, nuts and fruit as an excellent high-energy snack, or sprinkle them onto baking for a crunchy topping. Add them also to cereals for breakfast, and to put more crunch into toppings. Other calcium-rich foods include:

- gomasio – a mixture of sesame seeds and sea salt which is a good condiment and will also help you reduce salt intake. This makes a very tasty coating for tofu or chicken
- halvah – sweetened sesame seed paste which is hardened and cut into blocks. Nuts and honey are usually added. A very popular dessert
- tahini – creamed sesame seed paste that can be used as a spread like peanut butter and goes well with honey. You can also add it to cooking or eat as a dip
- green vegetables
- nuts
- dried fruit
- soya beans
- bony fish (the calcium is in the bones – think of sardines – when you eat the whole fish)

- parsley, dandelion leaves, nettles, kelp
- and, of course, milk.

Using soya 'milk' instead of cow's milk every day will soon increase daily intake, and switching from peanut butter to tahini will increase your calcium levels and make digestion easier.

Iron

Iron is key to having enough energy. It is the element in your blood which is able to carry oxygen around the body and deliver it to the tissues, like the brain, where it is most needed. We lose iron every month with a period, and it needs to be replaced. Lack of this vital mineral can lead to feelings of tiredness, increased irritability, and interrupted menstrual cycle. Foods high in iron include:

- egg yolks
- broccoli
- berries
- molasses
- soya beans
- whole grains
- green vegetables
- dried fruits
- cocoa
- wine.

B Vitamins

Adding B vitamins and carbohydrates to your diet will soothe your nervous system and help you manage stress. These vitamins will work to strengthen your nerves, and will also encourage good sleep.

Good sources of the B vitamins include:

- yeast
- green vegetables (especially broccoli)
- nuts and seeds
- whole grains
- eggs
- some seafood.

Fat

Reduce the amount of saturated fat in your diet (this is the fat that comes from animal sources) by switching to vegetable sources wherever possible, and avoiding deep-fried food. Being under stress means you are likely to sweat more, and this can leave you slightly dehydrated, so it is especially important to make sure you drink enough neutral fluids like water and dilute juices. This also helps bulk out the extra fibre you need to be taking, and will help move blood cholesterol out of your system and improve peristalsis.

When your body is under stress, it does not metabolise protein very well, so whatever type of protein you choose, you must attend to your body's need for regular, small amounts.

Sea Vegetables

Sea vegetables are excellent sources of iodine (necessary for a good metabolic rate and the ability to burn up what we eat) and are rich in a range of other minerals. You will find these in many supermarkets as well as specialist and healthfood stores, and they form a substantial part of Chinese and Japanese menus. These include:

- Nori – a deliciously tasty seaweed that can be bought in flakes for you to sprinkle on food, or in sheets. These are often used to make sushi, and you can wrap rice and other things in the sheets, roll them up, and then slice them, or toast the sheets until crispy and flake over a meal.
- Wakame – comes in longer strips that actually look something we might expect from a seaweed. Soak these for a short time and then snip into salads, or add to soups and one-pot meals.
- Kombu – a very good tonic and useful for helping rid the system of heavy metals. You can cook a strip with rice, or any soups or one-pot meals.
- Carrageen – can be ground and added to a meal, or used for its gelatinous qualities to make sweets, fruit jellies, and in place of aspic.

Mung Beans

This humble legume is invaluable for keeping the pelvis clear. It is good for supplementing oestrogen levels (excellent before and during the menopause) and is a rich source of protein. Eat the beans boiled up in water to make a soup or thin stew, and add vegetables, herbs and spices to flavour. Potatoes go particularly well with mung, as does cumin spice, black pepper, courgette and celery. You can also cook mung beans to a dry mix (letting the water evaporate as you cook them) and when soft shape and form into burgers. Do not add salt when you are cooking as this will make the beans hard. Split mung beans are also available which take less time to cook, and you can buy them as a dhal – with the green coats taken off. This cooks up very quickly and has a more concentrated and nutty flavour. Sprout mung beans (see pp100–101) to cook, and to add to salads. They grow in 3–5 days and are extremely tasty.

Oestrogen-rich Foods

When approaching the menopause, oestrogen-rich foods can be included more regularly in your diet. These include:

- sprouted seeds
- bananas
- oats

- soya in all its forms, including tofu, soya sauce and soya 'milk'
- mung beans
- alfalfa
- celery
- anise, fenugreek, sage, calendula, fennel, liquorice and ginseng.

Simply switching from cow's milk to soya 'milk' for all your hot drinks etc, will make a significant difference to your diet. There is no significant difference in the taste, and it is as versatile as cow's milk. Consider having a hot milky (soy) drink before bed to top up calcium and pre-oestrogen levels for the day and encourage good sleep. This is also a good snack suggestion if time is short, or you are not feeling too hungry.

Dietary Challenges

Allergies

When we are fit and healthy we are able to deal with minor irritations that come from eating foods that do not suit us, but when we are under pressure, or the body's resources are stretched, this additional load can be just too great. Sometimes food has a cumulative effect too, so eating something that is a mild irritant for twenty years may be enough of a load to break down our natural ability to cope with it.

It is quite common to have an allergy to foods, or an intolerance to them, and this can throw up a range of symptoms all of which will compound our feelings of being unable to cope, or of being under additional stress. Common symptoms include:

- headache
- low energy
- irritability
- altered sleep patterns
- bloating
- fluctuating energy levels
- food cravings
- indigestion and constipation or diarrhoea

Although sensitivities may be hereditary, many allergic reactions can be because of a breakdown of the body's ability to recognise or process a particular food substance, and this can be aggravated when we eat a lot of that food. Having been introduced to some foods as babies, before our digestive systems were able to really deal with them, may also set up a potential intolerance. One of the best health steps you can take when feeding babies and infants is to delay the introduction of wheat and dairy produce. These are often given far too early, before we have the digestive enzymes and ability to cope with them.

Cow's milk is really an excellent food for calves. A

surprising number of people are allergic to milk protein. It is high in cholesterol and a large intake is associated with an increased risk of heart problems. Milk sugar is digested in the stomach by an enzyme called lactose, and we stop producing that enzyme after about five years of age. Contamination of milk products with hormones, antibiotics and other agricultural chemicals can produce adverse reactions, and the effects of pasteurisation on the chemical structure of milk are all yet to be fully understood in terms of their impact upon our health.

When we eat specific foods that have chemicals bound to them that the body cannot recognise we may also cause allergic reactions, and although the reaction will be to the chemical it will be masked by the food. Working out what foods irritate you can involve some detective work, but it is well worth it. Identifying personal allergens is one of the ways to maximise our positive nutrition, and will enable us to ensure that we focus the body's resources on optimum performance.

If you are keeping a diet diary (see pp109–11) in order to balance your everyday diet, it will be easier to spot any problem foods or food groups. Of particular benefit will be your notes on your emotional as well as physical well-being after eating. If you suspect you are having a problem with a food, keep the diary for a full month to confirm your findings. You may like to review it with a natural healthcare practitioner to confirm your findings and get professional advice on tailoring your diet to avoid those foods, and balance it with other sources of nutrition.

As mentioned already, wheat and dairy foods are among the most common causes of problems, but you could be allergic to anything – or your system could just be overloaded and reacting erratically to less than optimum nutrition or regularity of meals. If you can identify a problem food, give yourself a rest from it for one month, and you will notice an improvement in your energy levels, enhanced digestion, and relief from many niggling health symptoms. This is almost guaranteed. To do this successfully, though, you will need to be vigilant about what and where you eat, and read labels on all packaged foods. Wheat, for instance, crops up in a multitude of surprising places, including as a dusting on potato crisps, as a filler in sauces, as part of the batter around fish and vegetables, and in rye and other breads, noodles and pastas.

Look out for good alternatives so that your diet is rich and varied during this month. If you are avoiding dairy foods, you might try soya 'milk', cheese and yoghurts, and the range of 'milks' made from rice, oats, nuts and seeds. Butter seems to be the most well tolerated dairy food, although if you want to avoid this too, choose olive oil and use sunflower oil for cooking, and resist using margarines whatever their main ingredient. The chemical processes that render the fat spreadable are long and complex. Hydrogenating the fat radically changes its chemical composition and produces a less than beneficial effect within the body, rendering much of the nutrition inaccessible and increasing the amount of free radicals in your system. (Free radicals are agents that are responsible for cell damage, and which contribute to the ageing process, generating a high degree of internal stress.)

If you are avoiding wheat, look to add corn, oats, millet, rye, potatoes, quinoa, amaranth, buckwheat and soya as grains, flours, etc.

Do not eliminate more than two foods or food groups from your diet without professional advice to ensure you do not experience any nutritional deficiencies.

Food Cravings

Food cravings can appear at any time and may be a response to nutritional deficiency in the diet. They are common before a period, when they may be a sign of low energy, or during pregnancy. The mechanism of muscle contraction is dependent upon a fairly precise sodium/magnesium balance, and this is why salt cravings often appear when a period is due. Muscle contractions also occur, of course, when we are stressed in other ways – either from additional internal stresses or by external factors, or, as is most usual, by a combination of both. Meet cravings for salt by drinking less that day, and increase the fresh fruit and vegetables you eat to increase a balanced intake of both natural sodium and magnesium. Cravings for chocolate can mask a need for iron and this is essential for us to have the energy we need for everyday life.

Chart your own cravings, and also any swing in taste desires from savoury to sweet, and see how these change over your monthly cycle and in relation to the amount of stress you are experiencing day to day. Endeavour to meet dietary needs early in your cycle to relieve symptoms of PMS, and use food clues also as an immediate answer to when you are feeling stressed.

Eating Disorders

Anorexia nervosa and bulimia are eating disorders that commonly affect women. They can manifest for a number of reasons, and often nobody seems to know exactly why, but there are strong links to the emotions, especially repressed unhappiness, unacknowledged stress and abusive situations from the past. Taking in nourishment is an engagement with life, and rejecting that nourishment is a symptom that something is deeply wrong. They are always life-threatening and need to be taken seriously. What characterises them as so important is that they seem to have a very rapid onset, and then quickly reach a stage which can be very difficult to treat.

Eating unhealthily and being unfit means you will not be as likely to manage your stress levels effectively. Some simple measures can help, such as keeping a diet diary to spotlight what is actually eaten and to check for any possible food allergies that can be aggravating the system. Maximum benefit can be gained from knowing that there are others in the same situation so that loneliness and isolation do not compound the problem, and self-help groups can be extremely supportive and encouraging.

Our bodies are remarkably responsive, and once they learn from us what we want of them, they will go on to continue that activity without our having to be consciously aware of it. So it is that after vomiting up food soon after eating on a number of occasions, the body will start to do this automatically. Retraining it then to retain food can be a lengthy process. Similarly when we ignore our natural appetite the body stops preparing for food, and if we regularly overeat digestion is impaired. These can also take some time to correct.

Restoring balance to a system that is upset in this way requires constancy and calm. Making mealtimes peaceful, and ensuring that the quality and purity of foods is paramount will enable a great deal of relaxation. Making mealtimes regular events, and sticking to a fixed timetable for them will also let the body relax into the knowledge that good, safe food energy will be available regularly. Foods that settle the system include long, slow-cooked meals and soups that are easy to digest as well as being nutritious. Try to avoid stimulants of all kinds, and even the energy rush of stir-fried and other quick-cooked meals, and stimulating spices such as mustard and black pepper may need to be minimised. Avoid sugar, caffeine and other drugs such as tobacco and alcohol, although a small glass of wine with food will encourage appetite and digestion. Make sure that chemical additives, preservatives, colourants, and all E numbers have the smallest place in your diet.

Consider approaching the psychological and emotional aspects of an eating disorder with a professional counsellor, healer, or therapist of some kind. Separating your body image from wider issues will help. Eating disorders are a very loud cry for help, and often dealing with any difficult or suppressed feelings with the aid, support and encouragement of a competent and caring practitioner will lead towards recovery and the restoration of full health. You can also get further professional advice about food properties and what your body's energy needs are from a nutritionalist.

Making Change

Making change can be stressful in itself. We all know many of the changes we might make to let food play a more health-giving role in our lives, but it can be daunting to consider finding out more about nutritional values, and giving up things we like, and substituting new tastes and flavours. A good rule is to take things slowly – you don't have to revolutionise your eating habits overnight to make them healthier and more stress-relieving. Taking things slowly may help relieve the stress of changing your diet and decrease the pressures in your life as well as helping you meet challenges with renewed vigour and energy.

Consider looking at one area of your diet – perhaps you add too much salt to your food, or eat too much refined sugar, or drink too much coffee or caffeine-rich soft drinks. If you have four cups of coffee each day, cut it down by $1/4$ and have just three. If you have two spoons of sugar in your tea, cut down by $1/4$ to having $1^1/_2$ spoons. See how this works for a week or so, and then cut down by another $1/4$. Similarly, you can add one extra vegetable to your meals, or eat one extra piece of fruit each day, and build up good habits that way. This is an especially good approach when you are cooking for and feeding other family members, so that you can all adjust together.

Substitution Table

Reduce:	In favour of:
refined foods, eg white flour,	whole-grain products
white bread	wholemeal bread, rye bread, sprouted loaves, rice cakes, corn crackers, rye crispbreads, etc
white pasta	wholemeal pasta, corn, rice, and buckwheat noodles
sugar	raw cane or muscovado sugar, honey, date syrup, molasses, fruit concentrates, maple syrup

coffee	chicory and other grain-based substitutes, decaf
tea	herbal teas and tisanes, warm fruit drinks, dilute fruit juices and concentrates
salt	fresh and dried herbs, spices and Gomasio

Chapter 5 – Other Body Needs

Beyond the essential care that comes from optimum nutrition, the body has other needs which can be satisfied to achieve a greater sense of balance. More specifically, these can help us find outlets for the build-up of energy that the stress response produces, and then assuage its effects.

Exercise

This is a lovely way to feel your body and enjoy its abilities, as it moves through the air in the way it is supposed to. It is especially helpful for those of us who hold our stress physically, locking into the muscles and holding ourselves rigid in places or habitually adopting stress-filled postures. Doing the body scan (pp45–6) will help to make you aware of whether you do this. Movement and exercise will relieve the immediate pressures and over time it also increases your general fitness and reduces your susceptibility to the negative effects of stress. This means that you receive double benefits every time you exercise.

As a Stress-buster

Any kind of physical exertion will let us burn off steam and makes for a fast-acting and effective stress-buster. It makes good sense to use it to balance periods of intense concentration or inactivity. When we exercise in response to stress, we use the heightened and increased abilities that the first or alarm stage of our stress response makes available to us in a positive way. Expressing or releasing our energy means there is less likelihood of us having to deal with the resultant frustration of inaction. It also makes it easier on the body – the mechanical pumping caused by movement helps clear the system of toxin chemical by-products, and movement gets rid of the high levels of circulating blood fats and glucose, and returns blood clotting ability to normal levels.

If you can't get out for a walk, then run up and down stairs or step on and off a low stool or a large telephone directory for a few minutes. Do some shadow boxing, kick boxing, or practise handstands and tumbles if you are fit enough.

Long-term Benefits

In the longer term, exercise is essential to good health. It restores good feelings through the release of endorphins in the brain, increases the strength of the heart and lung capacity, thereby increasing the heart's ability to deal with the negative effects of stress and also raising stress thresholds. Regular exercise changes the body's metabolism and helps lower overall blood cholesterol levels while maintaining good levels of the high density lipids that are thought to give protection against heart disease. Other physiological benefits include improved circulation because more blood is pumped around the body, and a better posture and greater strength from improved muscle tone. Digestion will be improved by the increased blood supply, and this helps maximise physical energy and redress the digestion-dampening effects of the stress response.

The more you exercise (within moderate limits), the greater the circulating levels of feel-good chemicals in your blood that will help you cope with mounting pressures, and the less likely you are to have to deal with the ongoing stress of frustration and resentment. Any type of physical movement counts as exercise, but to be really beneficial you need to:

- enjoy it
- do it regularly
- keep on doing it.

Exercises can be split into those that encourage stamina or endurance, and those that increase flexibility and strength. They need to have some aerobic effect, which means they will increase your oxygen intake, improving your lung's capacity and the rate at which your heart can pump. Both types of exercise are useful in combating stress.

Choose things that you enjoy doing, and you are more likely to keep on doing them. You can combine your exercises, or switch around and do lots of different things so that you do not become bored. Good exercises to increase your aerobic capacity include swimming, cycling and aqua-robics. There are tremendous feelings of power and satisfaction to be had from working out using weights in a gym and there is a great deal of fun to be had in reaffirming your sexuality and going to a salsa class. Alternatively, walking the dog will allow you to stamp out any of the frustrations that have built up through the day, as well as providing some fresh air. You need to know your own needs, and whether exerting yourself physically is the best way for you to let off steam. Over-training can cause its own stress-related problems. It can lead to exhaustion, obsessive attachment – when you transfer your emotional need or nervous energy on to the exercise – and will also make you more vulnerable to injury. So you also need to know your own limits.

Monitoring Your Pulse Rate

Check your pulse rate when doing aerobic exercise especially, and be careful not to exceed the maximum rate indicated in the table below. You can take your pulse easily by using your index and middle finger to hold the pulse point on the front of the wrist of your other hand, or find your jugular pulse in the front of your neck just under your chin.

Maximum pulse rate during exercise

Age	Unfit	Fit
20 years	140	170
30	130	160
40	120	150
50	110	140
60	110	130
70	90	120

Exercise physiologists recommend that for maximum aerobic benefit you need to train at a level of between 70–80 per cent of your maximal heart rate for at least 20 minutes three times a week to see optimum benefits. To determine your maximal heart rate subtract your exact age from 220, and then work out 70–80 per cent of that as your optimal range. If you are 40 years old, for example, your maximal heart rate would be 180, and your training range would be between 126 and 144 beats per minute.

Your pulse should return to normal soon after you

stop exercising. If you are quite fit this should happen within a minute or two, but may take longer if you are not used to exercising.

Getting Started

If this is the case and you want to begin an exercise regime, start slowly and prepare for the change this will make to your lifestyle. Begin with walking for 20 minutes at a time. This is enough to be a good workout and should be easy enough to fit into your day. Endeavour to do this on six days each week. Once you reach this target, increase it by five minutes each day until you can walk comfortably for 40 minutes. Don't over-exert yourself. You should be able to carry on a conversation while you are walking, so don't push yourself too hard. Taking shorter steps will work the muscles in your bottom more, and keeping your arms bent at the elbow as though you were running will increase your aerobic benefits. Keep your head up, but not so stiffly that you encourage any tension in your neck and shoulders, and always wear good sports shoes that are designed to give you extra protection.

You can increase the level of activity you generally take in small but significant ways alongside whatever exercise programme you are enjoying. Choose one of these activities for a full week, and build on your successes by introducing a new one every week:

- getting off the bus or train a stop earlier and walking to your destination
- always taking the stairs rather than a lift or the escalator
- practising isotonic exercises (see p67) when sitting for more than an hour at a time
- delivering any local letters yourself rather than using the mail
- walking short distances rather than driving
- planning evenings out that include physical activities like dancing or bowling
- joining in with the children's games like playing ball.

Weight-bearing Exercise

Weight-bearing exercises are very important because they will help us maintain the bone density that we need as we grow older. One of the changes that we experience at the menopause is a lowering of bone density, and regular weight-bearing exercise will reduce its effects. Placing repeated stress on the bones, and their muscle and ligament attachments, actually encourages new growth.

Putting one foot in front of the other really is one of the simplest but most beneficial forms of exercise. You can walk just about anywhere – whether it is in beautiful countryside, or up and down your hallway. Walking burns up as many calories mile on mile as running, and will have a host of knock-on benefits such as raising your metabolism and improving the rate at which your body burns off fat. Walking also wakes up your mind and improves the way your body-mind link works. Women who walk generally have stronger bones than women who do not, but gentle walking takes a long time to produce these positive effects. Better and faster improvements in bone density can be achieved by brisk walking, jumping or skipping (on a mini trampoline if possible), dancing on a correctly sprung floor, and through the stop-start activity achieved in games such as netball, tennis and badminton, and in fencing, judo and some other martial arts. Jogging can be good too, but needs to be performed with great care to avoid causing other health concerns. Jog on good surfaces with a lot of give, such as sand, grass or tarmacadam, to avoid jarring the joints of the spine, and wear proper running shoes with additional shock-absorbing insoles to prevent foot and lower leg injuries. Wear a well-fitting sports bra and consider having professional advice on good jogging and running postures before you begin. You will also need to be sure to warm up carefully before jogging to minimise complaints such as shin splints, and then wind down fully afterwards.

Muscle-strengthening Exercise

Strengthening our muscles becomes more and more important as we grow older – and this means paying attention to it in our twenties! Simple resistance exercises will strengthen the muscles very quickly, but need to be kept up if the muscle fibre is to remain. The benefits of taking up some form of strengthening exercise are legion and include having a positive effect on bone density, just like weight-bearing exercise does, so the ideal exercise routine includes both types. Although weight training and bodybuilding may seem a bit daunting, you can do this quite easily at home using strap-on weights and dumb-bells, or even cans from the kitchen. Do make sure that you know which muscles you are working with each exercise to maximise the benefits and minimise risk. The best way to do this is from a session with a qualified instructor, or by carefully following the directions in one of the many good books on the subject (see Resources).

Work at this at home by using a can of soup or bag of rice in each hand as you begin toning your upper body, and this will also increase the weight you carry and strengthen your legs. Careful sit-ups and 'crunch' exercises will strengthen your abdominal muscles. Whenever you are working on increasing muscle size or tone, remember to:

- warm up properly before starting
- visualise the desired effect – this will increase the effectiveness of the exercise enormously
- stretch out the muscles carefully afterwards.

Rest and Renewal

In order to benefit from the long-term effects of exercise, it must be balanced with periods of rest and renewal when muscles can repair themselves, and the body can integrate change. As part of a response to stress, rest – especially quality rest such as sleep, relaxation and meditation – is essential.

Sleep

Our immune system functions better under para-sympathetic nervous control, and this is most active when we are sleeping or experiencing deep relaxation. During the deeper levels of sleep, many immune functions are greatly increased.

Stress is a major cause of sleep disturbance – high levels of activity-stimulating hormones keep the brain active as well as the body – and not getting enough sleep means stress levels will be heightened, so it is important to cultivate a good sleep pattern for both long-term and short-term benefit. Our needs for sleep change throughout the month. We usually need more just before a period, especially as we grow older and this takes more energy, and we require more when facing challenges and high levels of stress. We are likely to lose years of sleep when we have children. The first few months when we may be feeding a baby through the night mean a massive change to our own sleeping pattern. Losing out on sleep means we lose both physical and psychological rest and renewal, and feelings of tiredness, inability to concentrate, and having lost out on dreaming can soon lead to other negative signs of stress.

Get to know your own sleep patterns and needs – some of us manage fine on a few hours sleep, others need up to nine hours a night. If you experience difficulty in establishing a settled sleeping pattern:

- Set up a good night-time routine during which you wind down from the events of the day. Make a regular pattern of things that you do to relax the mind. Have a warm milky drink – such as soya 'milk' – before you go to bed, and avoid anything too stimulating or vigorous (see Food, p112).
- Tie up the loose ends of your day before you go to bed. Look at anything preying on your mind and aim for completion or closure in whatever way best satisfies you (see also Letting Go, pp186–7, and Setting Realistic Goals, p195). This will leave your mind clearer and help you experience a sense of containment in preparation for an easy night's sleep, and a new and fresh day following.
- Avoid taking naps during the day unless they are essential to keep you functioning.
- Do not drink coffee after 4 pm and limit other caffeine-containing foods and drinks such as colas,

tea and chocolate, and avoid alcohol.
- Do not eat a meal less than two hours before bed, but make sure that you don't go to bed feeling hungry.
- Make sure you get plenty of exercise during the day and are physically weary.
- Keep your bedroom as peaceful and uncluttered as possible.

Massage

Beyond physical relaxation, this can be a boon in relieving the physical aches and pains caused by tension or by exercise. Massage is often seen as a treat – and visiting a trained therapist for a professional massage can be a wonderfully rewarding experience. There are many different types of massage and other bodywork therapies that you can experience. Consider having a shiatsu massage to reach deep into your muscles and release any tensions there, or Thai massage which is more vigorous and energising. Ayurvedic massage can include a range of different approaches from dry massage by two practitioners wearing silk gloves, to the slow application of drips of perfumed oil onto your forehead.

You can enjoy the positive effects of massage at home, whenever you like, as a legitimate form of relaxation and a way of meeting a real physical need. Touch is a very important element in our lives. We respond very well to it, and can feel a genuine sense of skin hunger if deprived of it. The warmth and gentleness of caring touch can calm and soothe many of our cares. We use touch in all manner of situations, often without realising it, and any type of positive touch – whether from intimately gentle massage, close dancing, or stroking a pet – will considerably reduce both the immediate and the long-term stress we experience.

Massage is a wonderful way to relax your body, or someone else's. You can use oils that you have perfumed with essential oils or warmed to increase their viscosity and the ease with which your skin will drink them in (see Aromatherapy pp154–6). You can also massage dry to tease and gently stimulate all the nerve endings. It is almost impossible to remain tense or anxious and worried while someone is gently stroking and purposefully kneading away your stress.

Massaging Yourself

Every morning when you wake up, and each night before you go to bed, give yourself a small dry massage to relax you and reconnect with your body. Do an all-over massage if you have the time and are able, or just work on your head, face and neck, and your feet. Using the palms of your hands, just stroke your skin as gently as you feel is appropriate. You are your own best judge in this. Your morning massage may want to be a little deeper, and perhaps a little faster to stimulate your body and wake it up, whereas at night you may choose to use slower, lighter strokes to quieten and settle your energy. This will stimulate the nerve endings that lie just beneath the outer layer of your skin, improve your lymphatic drainage (the way that toxins are removed from tissues) and is also really comforting. Keep your movements fluid and continuous, and use your fingers on smaller areas. Knead gently where you feel your body is inviting you in, and stroke lightly over joints and other bony bits. Work with your hands together to create a rhythm that is soothing and feels good.

You can massage just about your whole body – it is just the same as when you soap yourself in the shower; some areas are more accessible than others and lend themselves to being massaged as part of your regular routine. You can focus on massaging your hands – either dry or with some hand cream. Start by making small circular movements around your wrist with your fingertips, then stroke down the length of your palm out towards the fingers. Work into the fatty pads on your palm with your other thumb and make more light circles around each knuckle. Lightly stroke each finger in turn, as though you are pulling the energy right to the tips of your fingers, and then go back and pay attention to each joint. Finish with some all-over gentle strokes. Massaging your feet is always very welcome as well.

Massage using oils takes just a moment longer to

organise, and is a wholly different experience. Here you can choose oils that will add specific benefits to the massage – almond oil to enrich your skin, olive to heal especially after exposure to the sun, sesame for its warmth, etc – and you can enjoy the rich, luscious texture of working with oil on your skin. Place the oil of your choice in a saucer and put it on the radiator or over a dish of hot water for a few minutes before you use it to ensure that the oil is warm and will be more pleasurable for your skin. Take a few drops of the oil in your hands and massage them together so they are completely covered, and then use this to lubricate your massage strokes. As before, work carefully, and use as much pressure as feels good. You can massage wherever you can reach.

Pelvic Massage

Massaging your pelvis is a lovely way to deepen your connection with yourself. It can form an important part of a retreat (see p208), and will help with a range of health concerns from pelvic congestion and constipation to painful and irregular periods. It is supremely comforting. Wait for 40 minutes after eating before you do this.

You can just use your hands to gently stroke your abdomen from your pubic bone up past your belly button. Make long, slow, sweeping strokes, moving in a circle up the right side of your body, and down on the left side. (This follows the line of your gut and will improve peristalsis.) Do not use any pressure, just let the weight of your hands provide enough. Feel as though you are really getting to know this part of your body, enjoying the texture and the warmth, and the smoothness of your skin. This part of your body is usually very soft and rounded.

If you want, you can use oil – chose olive, sesame or almond oil, and add two drops of an essential oil to add fragrance and health benefits. Howood is a woody, smoky-scented essence that is a good pelvic decongestant and will help if a period is late or you are feeling especially heavy. Rose is a delightfully feminine scent that is a strong uterine tonic (and needs to be avoided during pregnancy). Sandalwood is lovely for older skins and will support the kidneys as well as relieving tension. See below for further information on aromatherapy.

Finish this massage by resting your hands over your belly button for a few minutes and breathing slowly and gently as if you were breathing directly into this spot. Cover yourself in order to stay warm, then relax and enjoy the feelings, sensations and images that you have just experienced.

Aromatherapy

You can perfume the oil you use for massage with two drops of essential oil to bring their own special relaxing and stress-relieving benefits. Choose ylang ylang, a sensual smoky oil that eases nervous tension, sandalwood for its calming and relaxation properties, or one of the lighter, mood-lifting oils such as geranium or neroli. Howood essential oil is a powerful pelvic decongestant with a fascinating and evocative scent, and clove bud is deeply warming and satisfying. Rosemary will help clear your mind, and lavender seems to balance out the system, ridding mental cares and physical tensions. Lemongrass is very grounding and will help restore balance if you feel in a spin. You will soon develop your own favourites and find those essential oils whose aromas work to relax and de-stress you, and you can make your own blends to get optimum benefits. In the winter months, you might choose more stimulating essential oils like eucalyptus and cinnamon for their warming qualities.

Check the effects of whatever essential oils you choose to ensure you are not over-stimulated, and do not use any that are contra-indicated during pregnancy or on other occasions. (Clary sage for instance is a wonderful muscle relaxant with a lovely perfume, and it will both encourage sleep and have a positive effect on dreaming, but it should only be used just before bed.)

Rubbing diluted essential oils into your skin is a fantastically heady treat, but you can also use essential oils as a perfume to carry on their good work, in the bath and as a room scent. If you add them to a bath, keep the door closed so that you can absorb all the aroma without losing any on the steam. This is a wonderful thing to add to your evening ritual to help you wind down before going to bed.

Chapter 6 – What You Think

How we think affects how we feel, and our ability to feel in control of a situation will greatly reduce the amount of stress we experience. Remember, before the alarm stage of our stress response is activated, the decision is made as to whether we can manage the situation or not. The more we are able to view things from our own safe centre and perceive ourselves to be strong and capable, the less likely we are to be thrown off balance by events and circumstances. Cultivating strength and power in this regard means remembering who we are and staying in touch with our own inner resources.

The views that we hold about ourselves and the way the world works for us will colour how relaxed we are able to be in our everyday life. It is worth reviewing our own beliefs to make sure that they are as beneficial and positive as we would like them to be. Sometimes when we dig a little below the surface we can find that other people's opinions and teachings are more in evidence than we consciously realise. Most often the religious and political atmosphere we grew up in will have formed a large amount of our own basic thought patterns, and this may be the source of some inner stress now when the way we behave and what we believe doesn't correspond with that earlier template.

Our attitude to ourselves and to what we do is all important. When we hold limiting ideas about ourselves and our experience then we may be more likely to experience frustration and the absence of the stimulation and excitement of new things. What we believe to be true for ourselves is usually borne out in practical, everyday reality, so if we don't feel we deserve to be happy, it may take us a long time to let happiness into our life on a daily basis.

Our self-esteem is an area that will always benefit from some positive attention. It affects how easy we feel within ourselves, and forms the basis of our ability to relate with others, impacting on everything from the ease with which we feed and care for ourselves to how well we socialise. Feelings of low self-esteem and lack of worth are very common for women. For instance, we have a history of feeling a sense of shame about our physicality that can be hard to shift. But every small change we are successful in making augments our own personal memory bank of good feelings. Our society too generally undervalues and blames us for those things that make us unique and we may need to work hard to establish a solid sense of self that can help us decide how best to move forwards in our own life.

Positive self-esteem means we are less likely to become stressed in situations and relationships because we feel more able and capable within them. When we feel that we deserve the best for ourselves, we are less likely to compromise in our relationships and in the quality of the experiences we seek out for ourselves. We need a strong sense of self in order to be able to be honest with ourselves about our own feelings, and in our dealings with others, without worrying unduly about what other people think This can help us to say no and to resist bullying and manipulative behaviour from others.

We have a wonderful tool in our imagination. What we believe to be true, and can experience as being true by feeling and sensing it to be so, has a remarkable effect on us. When we imagine ourselves to be relaxed, the body lets go of tension, whatever the situation. When we bring our imagination to our exercise we increase its benefits enormously. For instance, when we exercise a muscle and visualise it increasing in size then the muscle actually grows faster. This shows that whatever is going on around us, it is our own inner world that really counts.

We can use the powers of an active mind to transform our everyday experience and revolutionise our effectiveness – by channelling our energy into positive support for our goals and aspirations, and using imagery, visualisations and affirmations to further augment it. These techniques are remarkably effective for achieving optimum performance and success, whether we are cultivating the relaxation response, or looking for a better reaction to interviews (see Chapter 5).

Imaging

You can use this technique now to focus on something that you want in your life – perhaps a calmer outlook, or happiness in one particular area. Make yourself comfortable – sitting is preferable to lying down so you are more likely to stay awake. Make sure your back is well supported and your feet are flat on the floor. Once your body is feeling comfortable, use your mind to imagine what it would be like to experience that. See yourself being that type of person, and relating with others in a new way. Flesh out your image in as many ways as you can, enhancing its reality by making it as true to life as you can manage. Create an image that you can hold in your mind, and colour in the background with a wealth of detail, down to the feelings, scents and sensations that are associated with it. Spend time with this image – first to get it right, and then returning to it as often as you can to enjoy it. When we connect our current status with our vision of what is possible, and travel repeatedly between them both, we create a structural tension that inevitably draws them closer together.

Saying Yes – Thinking Positively

A positive mental outlook will have a strong effect on your physical and emotional health. Every time you succeed in turning a potentially negative situation around, or in seeing the best in a given situation, or finding the bright side of life, you establish a clear pattern of positive thoughts and feelings. You can set up a memory bank that can shore you up when things get tough, and will serve to remind you of how good things can be.

As women we risk buying into the notion that we should always be nice and make the best of things – being the peacemaker and fitting other prescribed roles. Sometimes being nice means that we care more for other people's feelings than we do for our own. We need to champion our own feelings and learn how to express them effectively as an important life skill. Honesty is often much more generous to ourselves and to others than any type of compromise to embody another's feelings. Thinking positively really means learning to see the positive in your life, without necessarily changing the negative. This is not about denying your everyday reality, or any difficult feelings that you may have, but about finding another way to feel in control of situations and thereby minimise your stress response.

You can make positive choices for yourself at every turn. You always have choice and can use this to make very real changes in your life that will augment the quality of almost every moment. You can decide whether to listen to the bad news on the television or to some uplifting music on your headphones; to surround yourself with healthy, happy friends or moaning grumps. Choose to enjoy some physical activity most evenings, or become a couch potato; stretch your mind by learning new things and achieving successes for yourself or settle into a comfortable rut and warm yourself with your old prejudices.

Keeping an activities diary for just a few days will show you just how much time you spend without even thinking about it on things that do not necessarily further your own goals for yourself and your desires for your future. Consider how much time you spend watching television, surfing the internet, travelling to and from work, or chatting on the telephone. Over a week the minutes and hours all mount up. Imagine if you spent just one tenth of that time focusing on something positive that would bring joy and pleasure into your life in a new and exciting way. Ditching negative patterns of behaviour is as easy as replacing them with new, positive ones. Let your heart and your sense of enjoyment guide you. If you need to get up off the couch in the evenings, and want to take more exercise, see what you like doing – it might be taking long walks with your dog, when you can clear your mind and enjoy the relative solitude, or perhaps you like getting hot and sweaty in the gym, or prefer the social side of a salsa or ballroom-dancing class. If you need to give up some bad habit, perhaps having too much salt in your diet, focus on the positive side of experimenting with herbs and spices and exploring all those new tastes and flavours. If you focus on the negative you are left with feelings of deprivation and loss, but staying in the positive means enjoying the adventure of a new challenge. Being positive means seeing what it feels like to hear yourself saying 'I can', 'I will' and 'I do' more often.

Affirmations

Affirmations are a very good way to make sure that your mind is filled with inspiring, supportive messages that will encourage you in whatever direction you choose. You can use them to focus your attention on anything that you want to be successful with, from managing stress more effectively to attracting harmony into an area of your life. Make your own list of life-affirming statements that you believe to be true, or wish to be or have been true, about yourself and your experience. Condense this into a short motto or saying, making it as personally appropriate and as specific as possible. Rhyme helps a lot because it's easy to remember and fun. Repeat this to yourself whenever you remember. By repeating it as often as possible you learn to believe it, because new patterns are established in the brain and reinforced each time we reaccess them. Write your affirmations down so that you can read them too, and use them as bookmarks, or stick them onto your workstation or wherever you are likely to see them often.

Use affirmations to support you in very specific ways, or to achieve a more calm and relaxed outlook on life, or a greater opinion of yourself. Consider hearing 'I am enough, I have enough, I do enough' every time you listen to what your mind is saying! Other good ideas are: 'I am always in the right place at the right time, successfully engaged in the right activity' and 'What I feel is real.'

Feeling Safe and Grounded

How we feel about ourselves and the way we manage in the world can be the source of stress. If we really feel deep down that the world is a dangerous place, then our posture from the start will be one of anxiety and defensiveness. Most of us feel that the world is basically good, or neutral, and if only we could remember this more of the time then things would be easier. Sometimes this is only possible for us when we reach beyond the material world that we interact with every day and recognise some greater energy such as the natural world and Nature's own laws, or our spiritual sense.

Moving beyond whatever daily struggles we may face means we can drop self-limiting thoughts and feelings and stop feeding any paranoia that the world is out to get us. So when we have those days that start with laddering a stocking, missing the bus, leaving your notes at home, etc, we can use them as an opportunity to test our own ability to manage our stress levels. Seeing these situations as a gift may be stretching things a bit, but at least they can be put in a better perspective if we hold a more positive world view and experience the universe as loving and supportive of us.

When we feel safe and secure in our own energy, we walk differently – holding ourselves in a more self-assured and confident posture that feeds back by making us feel better and more positive in ourselves. We create our own positive cycle. When we feel better about ourselves our sense of vulnerability diminishes and our stress response is lowered because we feel more in control.

Learn some easy-to-use techniques to remind yourself of feeling safe and secure in your own energy. Use an anchor (see pp93–4) or do the circular breathing exercise (see pp58–9). Or try:

Drawing a Circle

Draw an imaginary circle on the floor in front of you. Step into it and stand comfortably, feeling the support of the floor below you and the containment of the circle of energy you have raised. Cue yourself to remember these feelings by holding your circle in mind and taking a small step forward.

Developing Roots

Stand comfortably where there is no one else around and you will not be interrupted for a few moments. Take off your shoes and close your eyes. Become aware of the soles of your feet and how they feel touching the floor or the ground. (This is a great exercise to do outdoors when you can stand on some grass or sand.) Visualise your own root system, just like a tree's, reaching right down into the earth below you and anchoring your there. See the wide spread of the roots and how far into the ground they go, reaching out for your nourishment and fully connecting you with the earth.

Breathe deeply and freely, and spend a few minutes just enjoying the sensation of being planted safely and securely on this planet. Let yourself sway a little, keeping your feet in place and feel the freedom that comes from being able to move whilst feeling fully grounded and secure.

Each time you do this exercise you set up a memory that your body will hold and you will be able to return to when you need to feel that sense of safety. The more you experience it, the greater and richer the resource you will be able to draw upon.

Standing Your Ground

Find a place where you will not be interrupted for a few minutes. Sit or stand with your spine relaxed, and take a few moments to straighten and relax it. Take some full and easy breaths, and become aware of your own core energy that runs up and down your spine. Now visualise the very base of your spine, the sacrum, and picture yourself with a tail that extends down and out from you, still containing your own energy. This magical tail is very special, and as it grows you can follow it as it stretches down into the floor below you, and on into the ground. Stay with it as it reaches on further and further down into the earth, travelling ever onwards towards the centre of the planet.

At the very centre of the earth imagine a small space where, if you look carefully, you notice a hook. Wrap your tail around your hook, at the very centre of the earth. Return your awareness to your body now and see how right and good it feels to be anchored so securely.

These exercises can also help banish any space-cadet tendencies, and are useful when we feel wired or have an excess of nervous energy.

Chapter 7 – Emotions and Feelings

Feelings and emotions are based in the body and their effect can be experienced throughout the system. They are intrinsic to our world, and to our reactions to stress. Knowing ourselves and our feelings is key to managing our own stress levels. It can mean an end to a lot of the internal stress we experience as well as providing us with clear leads about the way we express ourselves and manifest the early stages of our stress response. During the first or alarm stage of stress, the feelings and emotions we experience are very similar to anger, and the resistance phase may include feelings of resentment. Grief is common to the final, exhaustion stage. These three feelings, along with guilt (another very common problem for women) can be among the most difficult to contain, and the hardest to manage. Learning to recognise them will help us identify our position in the stress response, feeling comfortable or at least familiar with them means we do not incur further stress through additional fear or anxiety, and knowing ways to express them will diffuse the overall stress we are feeling.

Some feelings are easier to experience than others, and like any other skill, managing our own feelings is something we become better at the more we do it. Getting to know our own feelings is the first step towards allowing ourselves free expression – therefore making sure that we do not add to our own stress levels by clamming up when we would profit by speaking out, or bottling up feelings that need to be shared.

Bottling up the more negative feelings – like grief, anger, and despair – can lead to a hostile attitude towards life and other people, and may also contribute to depression and adversely influence everyday health. Often our feelings can seem bigger, scarier, or more destructive than they really are just because we are keeping them shut up inside. Sometimes letting out a shout, stamping your feet or crying can be enough to vent the excess emotion and release the energy, but if you find yourself needing to do this regularly, then there may be more effective ways to express and understand these feelings.

Getting to Know Your Feelings

Being at home in our own emotional world is a vital skill for women, and one that will significantly reduce emotional and physical stress. We tend to be very aware of the feelings and emotions around us, being able to assess and react to them whenever we notice them. Sometimes, if we are off centre or unaware, we can soak up the feeling atmosphere in a room just like a sponge, and this can cause considerable inner confusion. The more we know our own emotional responses, the more we are able to navigate these types of situations successfully. Consider keeping a journal in which to record your feelings. This can provide true insight into the range of feelings you experience as, often, having a safe containment for feelings allows us to express them more fully and to explore them more. Looking back over your entries can also give you a clear view of how things have changed for you over time.

Saying NO

When we are 'nice' – accommodating, putting other people first, being concerned about their welfare ahead of our own – this can make it hard for us to refuse other people's demands and requests, and can leave us feeling under-valued and tired. We can feel guilty if the people around us are not happy, and feel that to be our responsibility. Because we are usually very aware of the dynamics of relationships and the silent dialogues that occur between people, we will often be very keyed in to the emotional atmosphere, and able to sense what is needed in a situation to harmonise it or bring ease or resolution. In fact, we are often much more in tune and able to respond to other people's emotions rather than our own.

One of the hardest things for many of us to do is to refuse someone else's request or need. This is in part because we know how difficult it is for ourselves to ask for aid or assistance, so imagine it must be so for others too. It is also because if we stop being accommodating and totally responsive, then we step outside a very prescribed role, and into unknown territory. We might fear that we will not be liked very much if we turn someone down, and further that we could incur their active displeasure. Women who have any history of dealing directly with abuse, or who feel especially vulnerable in any way will often stretch themselves far in order to please someone, rather than risk drawing any anger or violence to themselves.

With all this potential emotion behind it, it is little wonder that saying no can be hard. The point that needs to be borne in mind, though, is whether you are saying no to some aspect of yourself when you say yes to somebody else. Never saying no usually means repeatedly denying some aspect of yourself, so in reality you say no a lot, but not out loud or to other people, just to yourself. That hardly seems fair.

If you have been saying no to yourself for a long time, you may realise the resentment and unfairness that you feel every time you sense you are being forced to do this. You might be saying to yourself, or to a confidante: 'If he asks me to work late one more time I'll...' and the sentence is usually finished with some fairly drastic action that states how angry you feel in no uncertain terms. The more you let this build, though, the less easy it can become to deal with the situation reasonably, because you will be very aware of just how much resentment you are feeling, and this can make you tense and worried lest it actually slip out. It also puts your body, and other areas of your life, under huge amounts of stress. If you find it impossible to state your case without bursting into tears or screaming, then the situation is out of hand and you need to address this seriously. Consider talking to a counsellor who will be able to help you steady yourself and explore your feelings. Assertiveness training courses can be helpful and fun because you can share your experiences with other women in similar situations, and discussing your feelings with friends is always helpful.

If you want to start asserting yourself more and saying no to unreasonable requests, then begin by realising that doing this is a very powerful action. It is a clear statement that you are a person in your own right, and that you deserve to have your wants, needs and feelings respected. It is a wonderful thing to do for your own physical and mental health, and could well be the key to resolving many of your stress-related health challenges.

Start by noting to yourself the people and situations in which you feel you are being treated like a doormat. Do you make yourself available to friends for hours on the phone, listening to them moaning about their troubles, longer than you would like to, or when you had been planning to soak your day's cares away in a warm bath? Do you just smile when your boss piles more work on your desk – even though you know you are working at your maximum? How do you react to people in authority who you feel are over-critical – your parents in law, for instance, or others you might like to please?

Once you are comfortable with the word no, imagine some scenarios in which you might like to use it. Run through them in your mind, and rehearse what may happen. At first you might be fearful or anxious about what others will say and how they will respond to you. Let yourself run through what is likely to happen – you might feel that saying no is an enormously huge thing to do, but it could be met with a simple okay. If you are not used to using it, then people are likely to be surprised when they hear no from you, so you may like to imagine some of the possible replies.

No is a very clear word that is not easily misunderstood. Anything you say alongside it will qualify or explain it in some way. Sometimes this can dilute the message, but it can also make it easier for you, so that you don't have to deal with the silence that may follow. If you think you could be comfortable with silence, then just say no. Otherwise, you might like to move the conversation along and offer other suggestions as a way of not having to explain yourself. Or you might find that explaining your feelings is the best way for you. Experiment with different ways of managing this, and see what feels most comfortable *for you*.

The next time your moaning friend calls you, you could say it isn't a convenient time or that you can't talk now. You could tell her you are sorry if she's having a bad time, and perhaps you could arrange to meet up for a coffee some time next week; or let her know that the bath is running so you only have a minute.

When you are able to say no, you can be much more discerning, and you may well feel that you have more authenticity about yourself. When you do say yes to something, you and other people will know that it is because you genuinely want it, rather than it being because you are unable to refuse.

Worrying about whether other people are liking you enough is just a waste of your time and energy. If you are yourself, and do your best in any situation, then what is there not to like? And if others only like you when you turn yourself inside out trying to please them, then they are not seeing the real you – and that is a shame. Letting yourself relax, say no when you need to, and asserting yourself generally will do wonders for your stress levels!

Expressing Feelings

To deny expression of our emotions is to submerge a vital part of ourselves, and this is an awesome decision to take. It is certainly not a thing to do simply because 'being emotional' is a pejorative label that has been applied by people who do not have as great an access to their feelings, or who are frightened of them. Some feelings are more difficult to experience than others, and this is especially true about those feelings with which we are not familiar, or do not feel easy with. These can be anything, depending on your own emotional make-up and history. Here we look at some of the emotions most commonly associated with the stress response, and they are also the emotions which are most commonly stress-inducing! The techniques for exploring and managing them can be used to make any emotion easy to cope with.

Anger

Anger is an emotion which we may experience differently to men. There may be strong familial or cultural embargoes against our becoming angry, societal ones certainly exist, and without role models to copy or be inspired by, it is even harder. Anger can be a difficult emotion to express because it is perceived as a positive, dynamic and aggressive force, and usually one that women fall prey to or have to cope with being on the receiving end of. Having faced explosive, violent anger and experienced the fear and vulnerability that this engenders makes many women reluctant to explore their anger further. It is also sometimes seen as overly 'aggressive' or unfeminine! When we stop and think about our lives and the injustices and difficulties we encounter every day, and realise that it may have been 20, 30, 40 years or more since we let out any of our anger, we can become frightened, or simply decide that it might not be wise to touch such a bedrock of emotion.

Becoming comfortable with anger means exploring it in a safe and comfortable environment, where we can just look at the feelings. It also requires us to have a range of effective and contained ways in which to express it. This can transform feeling angry into an awareness of the tremendously positive and powerful experience that it can be. When our anger is something that we are too scared to look at, little wonder that we think it will be too frightening for others to deal with, yet once we begin to explore it and see that it is just like any other energy, then we can begin to use it effectively in our lives. Using anger appropriately means letting it fuel us into achieving great things. It releases all the energy that we had previously used to keep our anger down, or to pretend that it didn't exist. When we become more able to use it to protect ourselves it can transform the quality of our lives in very real ways, it can even be lifesaving.

Anger that is not expressed will often be experienced

later as frustration and resentment. If you are aware of these feelings in yourself, you may be able to trace them back to situations or occasions in which you have been – for any number of reasons – unable to express your anger.

Managing Your Anger

The first and most important thing you can do when you start to feel angry, is to make sure that you stay in the present moment. This is the same advice as for managing the early stages of stress. The two are intimately connected, and as said before, managing one will beneficially influence your ability to manage the other. Staying in the moment means keeping in control of yourself and responding and reacting to what is real right now. Your anger will be effective, and you will feel better after expressing it, if you can use this powerful force like a spotlight – being specific and focusing it on the very thing that you need to. The clearer you can be, the more direct your focus will be, and the more likely it is that this will be a positive experience with a beneficial outcome for everyone concerned.

To enable this to happen you need to be clear about why you are angry, and what or who you are angry with or about. This sounds very simple, but it is important to have spent some time getting to know your own personal feelings so that you can distinguish between what is your own emotional luggage, and what is a reasoned response in the present moment.

Getting to know your anger in a safe way will help you see what type of expression you are likely to use. Exploring your anger can be fun, because the surge of energy that is released when you let go of these feelings can be a remarkably useful force for you to use in any area of your life. The physical relief will also leave you feeling lighter and clearer, and more able to get on with your life. Work with getting to know this aspect of yourself through writing down your feelings, thinking about things that make you angry, and seeing where you hold this in your body, and exploring your darker fantasies of revenge and spitefulness. Don't indulge yourself, just follow your trains of thought, and see what the outcome is. Look at yourself in the mirror and see what happens to your face when you become angry. Can you command withering looks, or do you frown and look close to tears. Some people go very red in the face as if holding onto their rage, while others go white as they concentrate their energy on keeping anger down.

You also need to look at your lifestyle, and see whether not having enough sleep, being hungry, and experiencing physical discomfort have an effect on your anger tolerance. Other factors that are likely to impact are your alcohol intake (more alcohol is likely to make you less tolerant), and where you are in your menstrual cycle. Energy peaks around ovulation and just before your period starts can make you quicker to anger and more unpredictable. This emotional aspect of PMS is one of its major identifying factors. If you notice this type of monthly pattern to your anger, or your ability to manage your anger effectively, then you need to address your hormone balance as well as your behaviour.

Of course, managing your anger is not all about going inwards and changing ourselves – sometimes getting angry is a truly good thing to do and it is a remarkably effective tool for change. It is important not to forget that point as we work on our own growth and development. Sometimes you need to shout at someone to get them to move out of your way! Take a deep breath in for a count of five, and then breathe out in a slow and controlled way for a count of eight. This will encourage your body to relax rather than tense, and will buy you a little thinking time when you can choose how you are going to respond, rather than just reacting to the surge of emotion that you are feeling. As mentioned earlier, the clearer you can be with your anger, the more productive it is likely to be in terms of helping to achieve your desired outcome. You can let people know how angry you are by telling them – 'This is making me very angry' – or by letting them know that when they do x, you respond with feeling y.

As we become more familiar with this emotion we can begin to realise that once we have the choice and the ability to express it, we also don't *have* to. Exploring other ways to express anger and use it for our own benefit is a very enriching experience. This is the sort of energy that can let you clean your house from top to bottom in less than an hour. It is the powerful surge of creative energy that will let you solve long-standing problems, or power your all-night dancing session.

Once you know that you can become angry, and that it is safe to do so and you have an armoury of different ways of expressing that anger, you can feel more in control and be more able to respond to everyday situations. Staying healthy and being in balance means making positive choices for your future, and being responsible for yourself right now.

Anger management:

- Remember that no one else can make you feel angry. It is your feeling, your emotion, so take responsibility for it and then you can decide what to do with it.
- It is important to stay in balance. Always being angry, or never being angry are both sides of the same imbalance, the ideal is to be able to express yourself as and when you choose.
- If you feel close to losing control, distance yourself or employ a time-gaining exercise (like taking a deep breath in to the count of five, and breathing out to the count of eight).
- Stay in the present – deal with what is happening right now, rather than past resentments, unfinished

business, or issues from the past.

- Seek resolution – endeavour to find some sort of closure where you both feel you have achieved something.

- Remember to wind down. It can take up to 20 minutes or more to recover from an angry incident. Give yourself time to do this, and make sure that you tie up any loose ends and settle yourself emotionally before moving on with your day.

Meeting anger in others:

- Listen to the other person. Try to remain calm and hear what they are saying – they may just be needing to let off steam, or they may have a valuable point to make that you can relate to and empathise or agree with.

- Don't take what they are saying too personally – they may be losing control and lashing out. Try to see it as a degree of their discomfort, or how disturbed they are.

- Try to mirror some of their postures or actions (if they are standing, stand too), and raise your voice very slightly so that it is clear that you are affected by what is going on.

- Maintain a safe distance between you – this is situation dependent, but the width of a desk in an office, the length of a seat on a bus, etc.

- Stay in touch with your feelings.
- Be honest – say if you are feeling frightened, intimidated or concerned.
- Apologise if you feel it is appropriate and will help the situation.
- State your case as calmly as you can without blaming the other person or trying to shame them – these will only escalate the situation
- Withdraw from the situation if you feel you need to for your own protection.

Grief

Living with grief can make it practically impossible to maintain an everyday or normal routine without the overwhelming nature of the emotion overflowing into our daily schedule. Having a time in which to mourn is vital to our survival and our ability to function fully afterwards. Often the deeply painful nature of this emotion is one that leads us to close down from worldly events and focus our energy more inwardly. The effects of shock are similar, and it can take care and time to warm ourselves up again and get on with the business of living our lives.

Grief is always extremely personal, and it is hard to make comparisons or generalise about it. The feelings can be devastatingly numbing and the experience will usually change us at a fundamental level. It is probably the closest experience we have of death, and can be very chilling. It can also be hard to let go of. Actively choosing to move on – to live fully and to experience joy and warmth again – can be difficult, but is essential.

Living with grief means expressing it – talking about it, and finding creative ways to move beyond the enormous hole that it seems to be. Mourning is a process that needs to be honoured in order to fully recover from our grief, whether it is in response to the death of a loved one, or the loss of promise contained in a miscarriage, or the recognition of something that we never received.

We must deal with our grief, otherwise each future parting can touch on that deep inner well of unshed tears, and leave us unable to cope and respond in the present time.

- Reaffirm life in as many ways as you can. Search out those things that make you feel fully alive and in touch with your body and your emotions.
- Find a way to accept what has happened. Realise that this is non-negotiable and plumb your own resources to enable you to find some peace, or reason, or whatever specific thing you need right now.
- Talk about your loss.
- Give yourself time to feel your pain.
- Don't even try to carry on as normal.
- Stay in close touch with friends and family.
- Find a way to move forwards and on with your life.

Guilt

This is a common emotion for us as women. It may or may not be directly connected to our stress response, but it often underpins many of our thoughts, actions and reactions. Guilt is generally a waste of time and energy. It is a powerful emotion that, along with shame, has long been used to keep us 'in our place'. When we feel guilty about having our own needs met, or too ashamed of our body to express ourselves physically, we deny something very important. We also lose out on life.

Feeling guilty means identifying with fear rather than letting love illuminate our lives and move us along our own special and individual path. It can be hard to understand our guilt if we apply any logic to it – it makes little sense for victims of violence to feel guilty or to accept that having a physical body could be a cause for shame. Other good sources for guilt are having emotions, and owning sexual feelings. Some religions would have us believe we are guilty for just being born!

Wasting our energy on feeling guilty just adds to our sense of powerlessness, and the greater the burden of weight, the harder it can be to get rid of. We must remember that the past is done, and let it go. The best way to do this is to be alert and responsive in our lives today:

- Develop a good antenna for situations in which you feel guilty. Avoid them as much as possible or work to change your own responses.

- Ask yourself what you are feeling guilty about (does it hide something else?) and use a releasing technique (pp186–7) to let it go if it is no longer useful to you.
- Stop doing things that you 'should' or 'have to' or 'must' but don't actually want to do. Review how much of your time is spent on 'should do' activities, and see what you can change. Lose these words from your vocabulary.
- Learn to enjoy what you do, and spend as much time as possible doing what you enjoy.
- Listen to the voice of your heart and follow its best advice.
- Don't waste your time with regrets.
- Don't use guilt as an excuse for non-achievement, and don't let others guilt trip you into being anything less than you are.
- Remember that other people's opinion of you is none of your business.

Releasing Stress

One of the best ways of releasing stress is simply getting it out! Talking things through with another person can be very helpful, especially if you choose somebody that you can trust, and allow yourself to relax and fully express yourself. It is useful to separate what you are feeling from your logic about the situation, so even if you can simply say 'I know it is hardly fair, but I feel...'

then you untangle some of the knots that can stop us from releasing this type of energy. Often the logic of our mind can act as a block towards allowing the feelings that are in our heart, and acknowledging that gives both aspects of ourselves some freedom.

Letting Go

Releasing feelings or old habit patterns that we have carried with us for some time is easier if we can make some form of ceremony or practical measure to reinforce our intention. These are some techniques for reducing the stress and the burden of living with things in ways that no longer benefit you:

- Immerse yourself completely in whatever it is that you are seeking to let go of. Give yourself a time limit (a short one) and indulge yourself completely – wallow in your self-pity, have a chocolate fest, or picture yourself as that small, powerless, crying infant. Get the full measure of the experience, and when you know it fully you will be able to make the choice to walk away from it.
- Try carrying an object with you all day and let it symbolise a pattern or memory that you are willing and able to let go of. At the end of the day, discard or bury it, and walk away. Be clear in your mind that you are walking away from that thing which you have identified with the object.

- Become mindful of your desire to be more contained and powerful in yourself. You can empower yourself, or you can give your power away to some event in your past or some addiction that has caused you pain, or at the very least doesn't serve you now. Make your decision.
- Get rid of anything associated with negative memories or the past. Give it away, throw it away, burn it, or find some other way to get it out of your life.

Panic Attacks

These are an all too common reaction to stress – especially to emotional stress. One person in ten experiences panic attacks at some time in their lives, but they can be remedied. They can range in severity from mild but frightening episodes when you feel shaky and unsure of yourself, to more full-blown and incapacitating incidents that include dizziness, palpitations and a real inability to function. They can occur in direct response to a difficult or challenging situation, or in seemingly unrelated ways. They are most often caused when we do not breathe well enough. The feelings are part of a chain of events in the body which include a change in adrenal output leading to alarm-stage, 'fight-or-flight' energy rushes. There is a strong link with depression, and anyone who suppresses their feelings may find that they sometimes just erupt of their own accord. Exploring your feeling world in a safe and contained way can be key to resolving these attacks. Other physical measures that you need to check include:

- lack of sleep
- excess caffeine
- neat alcohol intake, particularly spirits
- specific food intolerances, and/or not eating regularly
- incorrect breathing – hyperventilating and taking anxious, shallow breaths
- where you are in your menstrual cycle – the high energy of a late period can cause similar symptoms.

Being familiar with your emotions, and feeling able to work with them and express them in ways that suit you will help ease any on-going symptoms. Learning some good relaxation techniques that work for you will also work to help you resolve this. Make sure that you practise them regularly, and give yourself plenty of time for this each day. Learn some relaxation shortcuts as well as making time to fully relax at least once every day for a while, or until your panic comes within your control again.

If you experience a panic attack:

- Keep breathing. Keep your breathing full and

relaxed, and count as you breathe in each time to the count of at least five, counting as you breathe out each time to at least eight. Making each exhalation longer than the inhalation will help your body relax. Breathing into a paper bag for one minute may also help you to relax.

- Tell yourself that this has happened before and you have survived it. It will be okay.

- Occupy your mind by reciting a poem, counting backwards from 20, or repeating your own personalised reassurances or affirmations. Good affirmations might include: 'I am safe and warm and everything is going to be well'; 'I am enough, I have enough, I do enough'; and 'It is okay, I am okay.' They don't have to be anything profound, just reassuring, but the best ones are those which are personal and therefore more meaningful to you.

- Acknowledge your feelings – don't try to fight them. Endeavour to identify and name all the different emotions you are experiencing from fear and panic on to whatever else you are aware of. You can deal with these later.

- Loosen any tight or restrictive clothing – unbutton your waistband, or loosen your bra if they feel at all tight or constricting.

- Use an anchor or instant relaxation aid to help you relax physically (see pp93–4).

Chapter 8 – Other Life Skills

This final chapter looks at other vital ways to look after yourself and plan your life.

Relationships

We all need to experience love and support in our intimate relationships and also in the passing kindnesses we receive and the respect of colleagues and acquaintances. It is key in preventing a predisposition to stress (see Chapter 1) and influences how well we are able to withstand the pressures of long-term stresses. When we feel secure and loved, our circulating levels of noradrenaline, adrenaline and cortisol are all normal.

You are in relationship with everything around you, from the air you breathe, to the people you smile at when you meet, and the pets you have in your home.

When you acknowledge that great sense of connectedness, you are able to relax and lose many worries and individual cares. Simply being loving, even if it is just in the space of your own home, or with your pet, reduces your stress levels because it allows you to manifest a vital and central aspect of yourself. When you can act from this place within yourself, your relationships are less likely to be stressful and strained.

Each loving, positive thought that you have towards yourself and others, every kind gesture and generous act of forgiveness, fills *your* experience with a sense of balance and harmony. Loving yourself means eating well, making sure you are safe and happy, giving yourself time for fun and pleasure, and to deepen your understanding of your own motivations and feelings.

The way we relate to others is an important aspect of our own stress levels, and a measure of how successful we may feel in our life. Most of us encounter stress in an area of our relationships at some time or other. Often they can be situations or patterns of relationship that repeatedly occur. Think about what happens, what your typical stressed response is, and about why you think it affects you that way. Among your range of responses you may need to begin charting those which are most effective at relieving the stress of the situation. Ask yourself the following:

- Is it only in *that* relationship that I always respond

in a certain way or is it common to all my dealings with people?

- What common areas can I see? For instance, is respect an issue for me? What about self-worth? Do I move to accommodate other people's feelings without making space for my own?
- Does it matter how close people are – is it only with those closest to me that I will react a certain way? Sometimes we can only be angry with people with whom we feel safe, or we cannot orgasm within an established relationship.
- Are there certain things I hear that set me off, or certain physical situations? For instance, is it every time I hear someone say that I am over-reacting, or whenever I am driving and the passenger starts telling me where to go?

Review your day from a relationship standpoint, and see how effective or stressful your communications were. Analyse them to see which were successful, and why, and which are providing you with areas to grow and learn. Good strategies in relationships include:

- saying, honestly, 'when you say/do *that* it makes me feel...'
- taking a moment to ask yourself if you think the other person *means* to insult or offend or irritate you, or whether they are just upset

- expressing your positive feelings often – being loving, appreciative, generous and congratulatory
- moving physically. This will alter your exchange and may be enough in itself to redress any imbalance. It will also relieve your physical tension if you are holding on to feelings.

Asking For Help

One of the easiest ways to relieve stress can be to ask for help, but this can often be hard to do. Sometimes we need aid or assistance with something, but feel too vulnerable or needy to ask for it reasonably. It can seem as though our need for support is so great, that if we tell someone that we aren't able to work our account, or open a file, or put up a shelf, then we are really letting them see the depth of inadequacy that we are feeling inside. Not being able to cope with the pressures of our lives, or being poorly skilled in specific areas are not crimes. Letting people help us is often a very generous thing to do – many people derive a great sense of worth and satisfaction from being able to help others.

As with everything we say or do that can have an overlay of strong feelings, it is important to realise that we can keep it simple. We are aware of feelings, and it is easy to assume that everyone else is as well. Learning to say what you need is a great skill. Practise finding ways to ask for what you need. Be clear and simple – you don't always have to explain why, or fill in background details. Find one area of your life where you could benefit from someone else's assistance, consider the best place to look for help or the best person to approach, and go right ahead and do it.

- Work out what this help is worth to you. You may want to ask for it as a favour, and could consider what you might offer or be prepared to do in return, or you might want to have a fee in mind or suggest a barter. Maybe you could just ask for it as a gift of kindness.
- Consider how much thanks or gratitude is appropriate, and bear in mind the consequences – how this may alter your relationship, and how it will change your life.
- Prepare for rejection – sometimes people are not able to do the specific thing you ask for. It doesn't necessarily mean that they don't like or love you, or don't want to help in another way. Try to respond to any refusal in a practical way – have an alternative request in mind, or ask 'Why not?'
- Remember you can always change your mind – that means you can:
  - ask for more help, e.g. that was great, would you consider teaching me how to . . .
  - renegotiate the terms you have agreed if it doesn't feel right at any time
  - say that you no longer want that thing done or need their help.

Setting Realistic Goals

This can be applied to your hopes for a relationship, any other specific project, or to your life as a whole. It is all about organising and prioritising the task in hand, and making sure that you allow for your dreams, but it doesn't set yourself up for disappointment if they remain as dreams. Not letting demands or expectations outweigh your ability to cope means you will not experience stress about it. When we ask too much of ourselves, or keep hold of perfectionist attitudes, we can only increase our sense of disappointment when we fail to achieve what we set out to do.

Write down all the aspects that are involved in the project or whatever area of your life you are looking at, and start to assess everything in terms of priority. You can have any number of top priorities, it will only make your goal settling easier. Review everything on your page and give each item a rating of one for most important to five for least. Some of the things may seem too difficult to attain, or of no real importance, and you can delete them or move them on to another list for now. Once your priorities are clear, you can begin to set some clearly achievable goals for yourself. Divide your aims into a long-term plan and a short-term plan.

Time Management

You can never save time, but you can use it wisely. Managing your time effectively is a way to feel and be more in control in your life. It will allow you the space to head-off many potentially stressful situations before you encounter them, and will relieve much of the pressure from overloaded schedules that can leave you constantly running late and being disorganised. Managing your time effectively will enable you to prioritise yourself, your relationships, your work plans, or whatever you choose. If you can do routine tasks quickly, you will have more time to enjoy your leisure and linger over the more enjoyable aspects of your day.

Managing your time is also about the deeper choice of how much chaos you choose to allow in your day, and how streamlined and organised you like to be. Over a lifetime, a substantial chunk of your allotted span could either be spent in disorder or instead in doing any manner of other things that will support and pleasure you.

The first step, as always, is to take a thorough audit and see how you actually spend your time each day. Consider keeping a time diary for three days, and marking down how long it takes to carry out everything that you do. Include everything from talking on the phone to relaxing in the bath. Make sure to note things that all happen together – we often manage to do two, three or more things at once. At the end of your time audit, read over your entries. Separate your findings into categories – home, work, relationships, etc, or by people – and you will see just how much of your time and energy is spent on what things, and with whom.

Organising your time effectively may mean becoming a little less available to those around you. This might be especially relevant if you found yourself spending a lot of your time involved with looking after others – it may be that your time would be better spent organising a car pool, or making sure everyone in the family knows that you only make one dry-cleaning run each week, or producing a rota for making coffees in the office.

A good diary or wall calendar is useful if you fill it in as far ahead as possible, and in as much detail as you can. List making is another good way to make sure that you are not trying to hold everything that you need to get done inside your head. Be sure to make a note of all the things you can delegate, and to whom, and make this your first job on each new day. By delegating what you can to colleagues, children, your partner, friends and family you can make it an opportunity to include them more in your life, as well as relieving some of the time pressures you experience. Spending time together doing things can add a real quality to most relation-ships, and teaching your children to do more for themselves will help them become more adept and responsible. Good managers always delegate, so see this as developing another of your managerial skills rather than as needing help with something. This is another potentially strengthening and empowering thing for you to do for yourself.

Once you have set yourself something to do, work

rapidly and intensively so that you will be able to finish it in a set time. Goals can give you a sense of direction, and very real feelings of achievement. They are also good in carrying you through dull or tedious patches. Whenever you make a goal, take a moment to picture yourself in your mind's eye, and see yourself confidently achieving what you want. Make some general goals for yourself that will enhance your pleasure as well as your effectiveness in the world.

Here are some time-saving tips. Take a little time to work out some individual aids that will specifically help you in your day. Often the time you invest in thinking things through and organising will pay dividends in better working practices and the quality of what you do.

- Keep clutter to a minimum – keep your mind and your intentions as clear as your desk.
- Decide what to do with things as soon as they come into your life, and act on that decision.
- Put things away rather than putting them down.
- Always be true to yourself, because it saves time in the long run.
- Always do the best job you can – think quality, because it invariably pays off. (But avoid taking it to an extreme – practise the difference between focusing your attention on quality, and being a perfectionist.)

- Trust your instinctive reactions to things, situations and people.
- Don't waste time with regrets.

Changing The Atmosphere

There are many occasions when changing the atmosphere or the dynamic of a situation will benefit us. If there are places where you spend a lot of time, it may benefit you to keep the atmosphere there as clean and clear as possible. Feng shui is an ancient Oriental art of tracing the movement of energy through spaces and its principles can be applied to clear and harmonise your home, office, or any other area. Essentially it is a way of formalising our need for balance, and looks to ensure that each aspect of our lives has a place, or that each elemental energy is honoured.

Energy flows through and around us all the time. The place where you are sitting now and the land where your home is built carry their own lines of magnetism and earth stresses. The presence of underground water will influence how well you are feeling, as can the proximity of other energy sources like electricity pylons. Sick-building syndrome is partly about this, and the nature of the things you use and keep around you. Generally, natural fibres and materials are least likely to cause any excess electrostatic energy, or give off toxic fumes, and are thus less likely to cause any health problems or increase your stress levels. Some people are very much aware of our sensitivity to these energies, and can diagnose the harmony of energy in an area. It is well worth considering such a consultation if you often feel a certain way in a particular space. There might be one room in which you always feel less than positive, or you may think that your luck has changed since you moved to a new office.

Simple measures can help. Avoid clutter and keep surfaces clear, clean and tidy. This is especially beneficial in work areas. Keeping well away from large electrical appliances like washing machines while they are running, and regularly wiping down the area around your television and computer with a damp cloth will help reduce your exposure to static and negative electrical energy. Moderate the use of a mobile phone.

The logistics of relating to people creates atmospheres in all the unspoken exchanges that occur between us. Endeavouring to be as clear in your communications as possible clears the atmosphere around you.

Smudging an area with a mix of dried herbs is a wonderful way to cleanse and change the atmosphere of a place. You can do this outdoors, to clear your own energy or aura – the space around your physical body that you consider to be your own – or to change the energy of the room you are in. Choose a traditional mix of sage and sweetgrass, which you can purchase loose or in a stick form (this looks like a huge cigar and is very easy to use), or grow and make your own from the dried herbs. Soon you will associate the pungent smell of smudge with a sense of transition into another state of calm awareness.

After scent, sound is one of the fastest ways to influence the atmosphere. Choose the soothing sounds of your favourite classical or instrumental music, play bird songs or the sounds of nature, or your own favourite tunes to encourage yourself to feel comfortable and relaxed. This is a great way to wind down after any trying circumstances, or after a period of exertion.

Making your own sounds is a lovely way to connect what you are feeling like inside with the outside world. Singing, toning, humming, even groaning can shift energy blocks and noticeably change your mood.

Treat Yourself

Plan some things to do with the extra time and space you have found in your day. You will have your own ideas, but consider:

- pampering yourself with a massage, haircut, make-over or long aromatherapy bath
- meditating for 20 minutes to clear your mind and cleanse your body
- relaxing and doing nothing at all
- going for a long walk to reconnect with the weather, season and your locality

- visiting a comedy store or going to see a very funny film
- beginning the project you have always wanted to, eg start writing that book, learning to speak Spanish, taking deportment classes
- doing something utterly frivolous, like in-line skating.

Retreats

As women we share specific challenges. We share the internal, physical test of riding a monthly wave of changing hormones, and face similar external pressures because of our role within society. Our bodies are different from men's. Even those things we have in common – a mind, a heart, etc – work and manifest our distress in distinct ways.

We live in cycles that wax and wane, embracing change at every turn, and enveloping us in a fluid and often seamless motion that it can seem difficult to anchor within a working week, or to any straight-line logic. We have a real need to celebrate and rejoice in that which marks us as different. When we can feel good about ourselves and our experience, then our experience is a better one. The more able we feel, the more competent we are in managing the stress in our lives. One of the greatest wounds we have experienced is in the degradation and shaming of our menstrual cycle. It is what connects us in a most profound and powerful way with the natural rhythms and cycles of life and death. It impacts upon every area of our life – from our sense of attractiveness (the hormones we put out at ovulation attract men to us), to our energy levels, appetite, and clarity of thought, and it affects us every day in the changing hormone levels we experience.

Each month there is a time when we are most outgoing and active in the world. This is when oestrogen and other energetic hormones are reaching their peak. There is also a time when we become less interested in the world out there, and more attuned to our own inner needs. The actions of progesterone in the second half of our cycle focus us inwards. This is when self-nurture and care can be most replenishing. Almost all of the activities we undertake – from stress reduction techniques to personal treats – can be maximised by using them at the time in our cycle when we will be most receptive. Exercise as a way to express mounting stress levels and relieve physical tensions is often most useful in the first half of our cycles, and receiving a massage may be most beneficial in the second half.

The moon has long been used as a symbol of the changes we experience throughout the month. It affects us physically, exerting its magnetic pull on the fluids in our body (we are almost 80 per cent water), stimulating ovulation through its beaming night light (at the time of the full moon) and by its effect on our environment (as well as controlling the tides, water levels in plants rise and fall in relation to the moon's face, and fruits even ripen faster during different phases). Most of us ovulate with either the full moon or the new moon. The moon waxes and wanes through each monthly cycle, showing us all its faces – from the magnificent hypnotic power of its fullness, through to the hidden nature of its absence. It can be useful to recognise the full circle of our experience, and the validity of each of our 'faces'. See pages 83 and 84 for some exercises that specifically connect with this in order to regulate our cycle, or just to reinforce this connection.

Going on retreat can be central to our experience as women. I recommend them most highly. They go beyond a stress reduction technique, or an aid to relaxation, and are key to our identity as menstruating women, or women who have menstruated, and are clear statements of celebration of that. Taking a retreat may be the only occasion many of us have to really spend time in our own company, working out what is important to us, and enjoying our own inner direction and timing.

Planning a Retreat

This is not something that is easy or practical to fit into the world in which we live, but it is the single most effective way I know to honour our own inner truth. It is remarkably effective in engendering a change of feelings about ourselves, and will manifest improvements almost immediately in any symptoms such as irregular or painful periods. I also recommend it as an aid to fertility. Every one of my patients who has done this, without exception, has benefited enormously, despite whatever levels of initial scepticism, and many speak of its transformational nature. Your first retreat is as special a time as your first period, and for many women it marks the transition from bleeding being a pain, to honouring the flow as a blessing, and marking a time when we have access to our own individual and highly personal truth.

This is a wonderful way to ensure that we have time for ourselves when we most need it, and that we are not continuing in our everyday routine, and giving to others or caring for their needs, but making the space to replenish ourselves and look to our own inner needs. Marking some time and space for ourselves when our period arrives is a way to honour our own fertility. It has been used in different cultures for centuries, but is often corrupted and misinterpreted to become a mark of the taboo that surrounds our menstruating. There are still societies where monthly retreats provide an anchor for women – a place where they may come together to share their common experience and the potential richness of that; or a time to reconnect with their own most personal and inner selves in a solitary way. This alters the whole experience of menstruation, enhancing its natural power, and reinforces our own cyclic nature.

You can do this each month, and take as long a time as your practical schedule will allow, or you can do it as infrequently as you need to. Just doing it one time can be a life-changing experience. One of its major benefits is in allowing us the time to spend really listening to our own needs, and the space to manifest those. It doesn't *have* to coincide with the start of your period (you may find it easier to arrange a retreat at the weekends) but the best times are when your period is imminent, or while you are still bleeding. This is when you are likely to feel the most benefit.

Take some time completely away from your regular routine, and make the space to experience and do whatever it is that you feel you need in your life right now. That may be something as simple as rest and relaxation – not having to get up to the sound of the alarm clock, or to get family members ready and off to work or school. Or it may be a sacred inner journey of self-discovery that allows you to connect with your own truth and refocus yourself for the month ahead. Meditation and relaxation may form the basis of your retreat, or you may feel the desire to focus on your creativity and developing ways to express that. Freedom of movement might seem apt – perhaps you need to do some dance or some t'ai chi, or maybe you just need the freedom of being able to just *be* without having to *do* anything.

Think it through beforehand and plan your retreat

carefully. There may be many practical arrangements to be made before you can find the time, and clear the space. Ideally, plan for this to last for three days, although one day may be sufficient. You can do this with friends, and there are societies and groups who arrange and lead this type of retreat, or you can do it alone. It is my experience that this journey can most beneficially be made alone, especially for the first time.

Practical points:

- This is time for you alone. Do not plan social interactions or dealings of any type. Turn off the phone, and don't plan to talk to anyone at all. The focus will be on your inner communication.
- Keep the focus clear. This is not just a time to relax or veg out. Don't allow television, radio, newspapers, etc, to pollute this sacred time. Step away from your old habits and choose positive and beautiful things to bring into your environment that will enhance your experience.
- Spend some time in Nature. Connecting with the natural world and the season will enrich your experience.
- Forget artificial structures. Take off your watch and forget about your diary and the calendar. Plug in to your own inner sense of timing that will tell you when it is time to sleep, when to eat, when to go outdoors, etc.

- Plan this ahead of time to ensure that you will have the space and the privacy that you deserve. You can tell people as much or as little as you choose about your plans, but make sure that they respect your need for privacy.
- Have a store of simple foods that do not require preparation or cooking so that you will not need to spend much time in the kitchen if you do not want to.

During your retreat, spend some time considering what your period means to you, and how your body handles it. You might like to include some period-related treats such as the pelvic massage (pp153–4); pelvic breathing (pp84–5); or breathing with the moon (pp83–4).

Try not to have too long a list of things to do – you may find that you uncover a sense of your life's purpose, but it is better to simply allow yourself to follow your own inner guidance and do what you feel like doing at the time. Keep some body treats to hand so that you can turn your bathroom into a home spa and indulge yourself if that is what you feel like doing, or use the time for a health fillip by just eating fruit and drinking plenty of good water to cleanse your system. You may find that all you want to do is listen to your favourite music and go for walks. Each retreat is unique, and we are all different, so use this time in whatever way feels right for you.

Monthly Treats

Whether or not you can manage a full retreat each month, this is a perfect time to make sure you experience some real treats. These can be anything that you find nourishing and replenishing. If you care for others, just having someone else cook for you can be enough to mark the change. Or you might plan something more sensual, or exotic. Making a regular time to care for yourself each month will help recharge your batteries and make a profound difference to your energy levels. It will have a positive impact on your general level of arousal and you will reap the benefits in terms of an improved stress threshold throughout the month.

Consider some sensual, body treats such as indulging in a Japanese bath ceremony, where you will be cleansed, then soak in scented waters, and afterwards have an exquisite full body massage before being wrapped in towels and given jasmine tea to sip while you relax. Or visit a Bowen practitioner for a bodywork session that will transport you to a wonderful world of relaxation and reap the benefits afterwards of better joint alignment and freer movement throughout your body. Explore the wonderful world of water and book a Watsu session where you will be held and moved through the water by a practitioner who is experienced in undoing all your knots and let yourself and them float away. There are myriad options that you can

choose from, and you need not opt for a physical treat –
you might prefer to indulge another aspect of your
nature. What is important is that you choose
something.

In Conclusion – Bringing It All Together

In modern times, the role of stress is as a strong indicator of unhappiness and dissatisfaction – these are the things we now need to be saved from in order to stay alive and well. We experience stress when we are unable to respond to our own basic instincts, but a natural approach to remedy this is still one that we will respond to most easily and fully. Taking a natural, holistic approach to the role of stress in our lives and how we may best balance that is dependent upon recognising the integrity of our response – as multi-dimensional beings who may suffer stress, and be treated on any or all of these aspects of ourselves.

Stress is an extremely subjective experience. Different events, feelings and experiences will cause each of us to respond differently, because of the vital initial assessment about the stress process – our definition of whether we can cope. Everything that we do to increase our feelings of being in control and effective stave off another excitation of our stress response.

Simple methods such as cutting in when we notice the very beginning of our stress response and telling ourselves in our most authoritative and confident manner that we can cope, or to relax and let it go are amazingly effective. So too are all the life-supporting methods we employ, such as all the pleasurable things that activate our relaxation response and let us luxuriate in some of the pleasure of being alive. Sandwiching our stress response in this way between quick fixes and long-term strategies squeezes it into an area where it is both manageable and potentially beneficial.

Harnessing the positive power of stress means we can use the excitement, enthusiasm and additional energy we feel to pursue those things that we want to achieve, and to simply make our days more interesting!

Too many of us labour on under a daily load of pressures that we perceive as being inescapable, and pay the price in the long-term health concerns that are associated with ongoing exposure to stress. Making the change to a more relaxed and healthful lifestyle means balancing our expectations and the demands upon us with our resources and our ability to cope. It means making sure we prioritise feeling good and all the techniques that maximise that experience alongside our commitments and goals.

You can begin making that change right now. Take a deep breath, and as you breathe out, relax your shoulders and feel your tummy and breastbone soften as you release the pressure on your postural muscles. Start making small changes to the things you do, the way that you do them, and what is in your mind while you are doing them. Make your attitude your first priority, and then see how easy it is to alter your physical habits. Keep foremost in your mind that you deserve the best, and can be and achieve this when you are relaxed and fully responsive.

Resources

Further Reading

Al Huang, Chungliang, *Embrace Tiger, Return to Mountain*, Celestial Arts, 1988

Balcombe, BF, *The Energy Connection*, Piatkus Books, 1990

Chopra, Deepak, *Perfect Health*, Bantam Books, 1990

Cowmeadow, Oliver and Michelle, *Yin Yang Cookbook*, Optima, 1988

D'Adamo and Whitney, *Eat Right for Your Type*, Putnam, 1998

Davis, Patricia, *Aromatherapy an A–Z*, CW Daniel and Co, 1988

de Long Miller, Roberta, *Psychic Massage*, Harper and Row, 1980

Downing, George, *The Massage Book*, Arkana, 1980

Grant Viagas, Belinda, *A–Z of Natural Healthcare*,

Newleaf, 1977

Grant, Belinda, *Detox Diet Book*, Optima, 1991

Viagas, Belinda Grant, *Natural Healthcare for Women*, Newleaf, 1977

Hall, Doriel, *Healing with Meditation*, Gill and Macmillan, 1996

Hird, Vicki, *Perfectly Safe to Eat*, The Women's Press, 2000

Jutel, Annemarie, *A Woman's Guide to Running*, The Women's Press, 2001

Kitty Campion's Handbook of Herbal Health, Sphere, 1985

Law, Albert, *Practical Feng Shui for the Home*, Pelanduk Publications, 1995

The London Rape Crisis Centre, *Sexual Violence*, The Women's Press, 1999

Looker, Terry and Gregson, Olga, *Teach Yourself Managing Stress*, Hodder and Stoughton, 1997

McNeil, Delcia, *Bodywork Therapies for Women*, The Women's Press, 2000

Northrup, Dr Christiane, *Women's Bodies, Women's Wisdom*, Piatkus Books, 1995

Oxenford, Rosalind, *Healing with Reflexology*, Gill and Macmillan, 1997

Paungger, Johanna and Poppe, Thomas, *Moon Time*, CW Daniel and Co, 1996

Sams, Jamie, *The 13 Original Clan Mothers*, HarperCollins, 1993

Shuttle, Penelope and Redgrove, Peter, *The Wise Wound*,

Paladin, 1986

Sneddon, Peta and Coseschi, Paolo, *Healing with Osteopathy*, Gill and Macmillan, 1996

Treben, Maria, *Health from God's Garden*, Thorson's, 1988

Villiers, Jack, *Pain Relief Without Drugs*, Millwater Publishing Co, 1999

Zeuss, Jonathan, *The Wisdom of Depression*, Newleaf, 1999

Contacts

British Association of Counselling
1 Regent Place
Rugby
Warwickshire CV21 2PJ
Tel 01788 550899

Cruse Bereavement Care
126 Sheen Road
Richmond
Surrey TW9 1UR
Tel 020 8940 4818

Equal Opportunities Commission
Overseas House
Quay Street
Manchester M3 3HN
Tel 0161 833 9244

Alcoholics Anonymous
PO Box 1
Stonebow House
Stonebow
York YO1 7NJ
Tel 01904 644026

Eating Disorders Association
1st Floor, Wensum House
103 Prince of Wales Road
Norwich NR1 1DW
Tel 01603 621414

The Miscarriage Association
c/o Clayton Hospital
Northgate
Wakefield WF1 3JF
Tel 01924 200799

Relate (Couples Counselling)
Herbert Gray College
Little Church Street
Rugby CV21 3AP
Tel 01788 573241

British Massage Therapy Council
78 Meadow Street
Preston

Lancs PR1 1TS
Tel 01772 881063

Association of Reflexologists
27 Old Gloucester Street
London WC1N 3XX
Tel 08705 673320

European College of Bowen Studies
38 Portway
Frome
Somerset BA11 1QU
Tel 01373 461873

Anthroposophical Medical Trust
c/o Park Attwood Clinic
Trimpley
Bewdley
Worcestershire DY12 1RE
Tel 01299 861561

World Federation of Healers
Hozzard Lane,
Blackford Wedmore
Somerset BS28 4UT
Tel 01934 712957

Rape Crisis Centre
Tel 020 7837 1600

National Workplace Bullying Advice Line
Tel 01235 834548

National Phobics Society
Tel 0161 881 1937

For details of Belinda's confidential postal Advice Service, a schedule of her workshops, lectures and seminars on relaxation and natural healthcare, or to buy a Bioflow magnet, write to her at:

PO Box 13386
London NW3 2ZE
England
(email: Belindasras@hotmail.com)

Established in 1978, The Women's Press publishes high-quality fiction and non-fiction from outstanding women writers worldwide. Our list spans literary fiction, crime thrillers, biography and autobiography, health, women's studies, literary criticism, mind body spirit, the arts and the Livewire Books series for young women. Our bestselling annual *Women Artists Diary* features the best in contemporary women's art.

The Women's Press also runs a book club through which members can buy, every quarter, the best fiction and non-fiction from a wide range of British publishing houses, mostly in paperback, always at discount.

To receive our latest catalogue, or for information on The Women's Press Book Club, send a large SAE to:

The Sales Department
The Women's Press Ltd
34 Great Sutton Street London EC1V 0LQ
Tel: 020 7251 3007 Fax: 020 7608 1938
www.the-womens-press.com

Kay Douglas and Kim McGregor
Power Games
Confronting Hurtful Behaviour and
Transforming Our Own

For both those who bully and those who are bullied, *Power
Games* is a definitive look at the power struggles in everyday
life, from conflicts that take place within the workplace and
personal relationships to the behavioural problems of children.
Kay Douglas and Kim McGregor explore both sides of a conflict
in order to help you understand what lies behind such
disagreements and offer strategies to build self-esteem and
assertiveness while treating yourself and others with respect.
Drawn from conversations with more than 50 women, this
supportive and practical book demonstrates how to recognise
the dynamics of power struggles in your life and how to claim
and express your own power with integrity.

Self-help £8.99
ISBN: 0 7043 4474 2

Kay Douglas
Invisible Wounds

A Self-Help Guide for Women in Destructive
Relationships

All couples have power struggles and disagreements at times,
but there is a difference between a relationship with the usual
ups and downs and one that constitutes emotional abuse. In
this practical, accessible and supportive book, Kay Douglas
draws on the first hand accounts of over 50 women – as well
as her own personal experience – to demonstrate how to
recognise, resolve and recover from a destructive relationship.
With advice on how to work out what is really happening within
a relationship; how to clarify needs and feelings; deal with an
abusive partner; get the support we need; cope with the effects
on children; regain our power in the relationship or decide to
leave it; and how to heal, this is an essential book for all
women who have, or have had, partners who are emotionally
abusive.

Self-help £8.99
ISBN: 0 7043 4450 5

Delcia McNeil
Bodywork Therapies for Women
A Guide

This informative guide examines the numerous bodywork therapies available, with particular focus on their relevance to women's physical and emotional health.

Including:

Massage, Osteopathy
Hypnotherapy, Rebirthing
Traditional Chinese Medicine, Acupuncture
Rolfing, Alexander Technique, Pilates
Metaphysical Healing
Bioenergetics, Gestalt
Trager® Approach, Zero Balancing
Yoga, Tai Chi and more.

Delcia McNeil examines each therapy in turn, outlining which conditions it will help alleviate and explaining its theoretical background and philosophy. She also clarifies what to expect at each bodywork session and provides advice on how to find a practitioner as well as suggesting self-help techniques to try at home.

Above all, McNeil advocates a holistic approach to health and the body – highlighting the effectiveness of focused touch, non-invasive treatments, sensitivity and intuition.

Health/Mind, Body, Spirit £8.99
ISBN: 0 7043 4569 2

Annemarie Jutel
A Woman's Guide to Running

Beginner to Elite

Running offers today's busy woman a chance to make fitness a bigger part of her life with no membership fees, no travel, and a schedule to suit her needs. A devoted runner and registered nurse, Annemarie Jutel includes tips on how to create a personal running programme, nutritional guidelines, and information about injuries and their prevention in this complete guide to running for UK women. Full of diagrams, tables, photos and expert advice specifically geared towards women, this highly motivating book is a valuable tool for women runners of all stages.

'A practical and fun-to-read guide that will help us all become the champions inside ourselves'
Kathrine Switzer (first woman to run the Boston Marathon)

Health/Sport £8.99
ISBN: 0 7043 4722 9